Women with Epilepsy

A Handbook of Health and Treatment Issues

In this handbook for women, their clinicians, families, and friends, Martha Morrell assembles a team of experts to review the special problems faced by women with epilepsy. In many ways, epilepsy is a different disease in women and in men. Epilepsy treatments affect fertility, and can cause pregnancy complications and birth defects, but most of the available drugs have been tested on men. Moreover, hormone effects on seizures are of particular concern to women at puberty, at menopause, and over the menstrual cycle.

Many health-care providers are not informed about the unique issues facing women with epilepsy. This book, published in association with the Epilepsy Foundation of America, fills that gap and provides women with epilepsy with the information they need to be effective self-advocates.

Martha J. Morrell is Professor of Clinical Neurology at Columbia University and Director of the Columbia Comprehensive Epilepsy Center at the New York Presbyterian Hospital.

Kerry L. Flynn is Manager of Research and Programs at the Columbia Comprehensive Epilepsy Center, New York Presbyterian Hospital.

Women with Epilepsy has been developed in collaboration with the Epilepsy Foundation as part of its Women and Epilepsy Initiative.

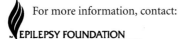

For more information, contact:

EPILEPSY FOUNDATION

4351 Garden City Drive
Landover
MD 20785
USA

301-459-3700–800-332-1000

www.epilepsyfoundation.org

Women with Epilepsy

A Handbook of Health and
Treatment Issues

Edited by

Martha J. Morrell and Kerry L. Flynn

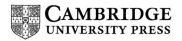

CAMBRIDGE
UNIVERSITY PRESS

PUBLISHED BY THE PRESS SYNDICATE OF THE UNIVERSITY OF CAMBRIDGE
The Pitt Building, Trumpington Street, Cambridge, United Kingdom

CAMBRIDGE UNIVERSITY PRESS
The Edinburgh Building, Cambridge CB2 2RU, UK
40 West 20th Street, New York, NY 10011-4211, USA
477 Williamstown Road, Port Melbourne, VIC 3207, Australia
Ruiz de Alarcón 13, 28014 Madrid, Spain
Dock House, The Waterfront, Cape Town 8001, South Africa

http://www.cambridge.org

First published 2003

Printed in the United Kingdom at the University Press, Cambridge

Typefaces Minion 11/14.5 pt, Formata and Formata BQ   *System* LaTeX 2_ε [TB]

A catalogue record for this book is available from the British Library

Library of Congress Cataloguing in Publication data

ISBN 0 521 65224 3 hardback
ISBN 0 521 65541 2 paperback

Every effort has been made in preparing this book to provide accurate and up-to-date
information that is in accord with accepted standards and practice at the time of
publication. Nevertheless, the authors, editors and publisher can make no warranties
that the information contained herein is totally free from error, not least because clinical
standards are constantly changing through research and regulation. The authors,
editors and publisher therefore disclaim all liability for direct or consequential damages
resulting from the use of material contained in this book. Readers are strongly advised
to pay careful attention to information provided by the manufacturer of any drugs or
equipment that they plan to use.

Contents

Contributors

Fariha Abbasi, MD
Neurological Center
900 Cox Road
Gastonia
NC 28054
USA

Janet Austin Tooze, PhD
Biometry Research Group
6130 Executive Boulevard
Suite 3131
Bethesda
MD 20892
USA

Elizabeth A. Borda
Women and Epilepsy Initiative
4521 Garden City Drive
Landover
MD 20785
USA

Mimi Callanan, RN, MSN
Department of Neurology and
Neurological Sciences
Stanford University Medical Center
Stanford Hospital
300 Pasteur Drive
Stanford
CA 94305
USA

Jeanne Carpenter, JD
McDermott, Will & Emery
600 13th Street, NW
Washington DC 20005
USA

Joyce A. Cramer
Yale University School of Medicine
VA Connecticut Health Care System
950 Campbell Avenue
West Haven
CT 06516
USA

Pamela M. Crawford, MD
Department of Neurology
Special Centre for Epilepsy
York District Hospital
Wigginton Road
York YO3 7HE
England

Patricia Crumrine, MD
Department of Neurology
Children's Hospital of Pittsburgh
3705 5th Avenue at DeSoto Street
Pittsburgh
PA 15213
USA

Patricia Dean, MSN, ARNP
Maimi Children's Hospital
Department of Neuroscience
3100 SW 62nd Avenue
Miami FL
USA

Aline T. Derdiarian
California
USA

Orrin Devinsky, MD
Department of Neurology
NYU Comprehensive Epilepsy Center
560 First Avenue
Rivergate
New York
NY 10016
USA

Yasser Y. El-Sayed, MD
Department of Gynecology and Obstetrics
Stanford University Medical Center
Stanford Hospital
300 Pasteur Drive
Stanford
CA 94305

Rosemary Fama, PhD
SRI International
333 Ravenswood Avenue
Menlo Park
CA 94025
USA

Kerry L. Flynn, MA
Columbia Comprehensive Epilepsy Center
The Neurological Institute
710 West 168th Street
New York
NY 10032
USA

Jacqueline A. French, MD
Department of Neurology
Hospital of University of Pennsylvania
3400 Spruce Street
Philadelphia
PA 19104
USA

Patricia A. Gibson, MSSW
Department of Neurology
Bowman Gray School of Medicine
Wake Forest University
Medical Center Blvd
Winston-Salem
NC 27157
USA

Dominic Heaney, MD
The National Hospital for Neurology and
Neurosurgery
National Society for Epilepsy
Gerrards Cross Chalfont Centre for
Epilepsy
Chalfont St Peter
Buckinghamshire SL9 ORJ
England

Andrew G. Herzog, MD, MSc
Beth Israel Deaconess Medical Center
Harvard Neuroendocrine Unit
330 Brookline Avenue
Boston
MA 02215
USA

Joan Kessner Austin, DNS
Indiana University School of Nursing
1111 Middle Drive
Indianapolis
IN 46202
USA

Allan Krumholz, MD
Department of Neurology
University of Maryland Medical System
22 South Greene Street
Baltimore
MD 21201
USA

Lisa Zobian Lindahl
112 Clay Point
Colchester
VT 05446
USA

Robert Marcus, MD
VA Palo Alto Health Care
3801 Miranda Avenue
Palo Alto
CA 94304
USA

Laura Marsh, MD
Department of Psychiatry
Johns Hopkins University School of
Medicine
600 N. Wolfe Street
Baltimore
MD 21287
USA

Kimford J. Meador, MD
Department of Neurology
Georgetown University Hospital
3800 Reservoir Road, NW
Washington DC 20007
USA

Martha J. Morrell, MD
Columbia Comprehensive Epilepsy
Center

The Neurological Institute
710 W. 168th Street
New York
NY 10032
USA

Ruth Ottman, PhD
Columbia University
GH Sergievsky Center
630 W. 168th Street
New York
NY 10032
USA

Steven C. Schachter, MD
Beth Israel Deaconess Medical
Center
Comprehensive Epilepsy Center
300 Brookline Avenue
Boston
MA 02215
USA

Philip A. Schwartzkroin, PhD
Department of Neurological Surgery
University of California at Davis
One Shields Avenue
Davis
CA 95616
USA

Patricia O. Shafer, RN, MN
Beth Israel Deaconess Medical Center
Comprehensive Epilepsy
Center
300 Brookline Avenue
Boston
MA 02215
USA

Paula Shear, PhD
Department of Psychiatry
University of Cincinnati
Cincinnati
OH 45221
USA

Simon Shorvon, MD
The National Hospital for Neurology and
Neurosurgery
National Society for Epilepsy
Gerrards Cross Chalfont Centre
for Epilepsy
Chalfont St Peter
Buckinghamshire SL9 ORJ
England

Jim Troxell
Epilepsy Foundation

4351 Garden City Drive
Landover
MD 20785
USA

Melodie R. Winawer, MD, MS
Columbia University
Sergievsky Center
630 W. 168th Street
New York
NY 10032
USA

Mark Yerby, MD
North Pacific Epilepsy Research
2455 Northwest Marshall Street
Portland
OR 97210
USA

Part I

The woman with epilepsy

Introduction: why we wrote this book

Martha J. Morrell

Martha J. Morrell is a Professor of Neurology at Columbia University, College of Physicians and Surgeons in New York City and is Director of the Columbia Comprehensive Epilepsy Center at New York Presbyterian Hospital. She has been elected an International Ambassador for Epilepsy by the International League Against Epilepsy and she chairs the National Epilepsy Foundation. Dr Morrell is the principal investigator on a number of epilepsy research trials examining reproductive health and hormones in women with epilepsy and bone health in women receiving antiepileptic drugs.

MJM

In many ways, epilepsy is a different disease in a woman than in a man. The differences arise because of biological differences between women and men, but also because of the different social roles they play. As a result of these biological and social differences, women with epilepsy face special challenges, especially in the area of reproductive health (Table 1.1).

The experiential differences between women and men with epilepsy became clear to me in the very earliest years of my career as a neurologist specializing in the treatment of epilepsy. My background had been in studying the effects of male and female sex hormones on certain types of behavior, so I was well aware of the significant effects these hormones could have on many brain centers. Therefore, I was not at all surprised when women with epilepsy explained to me that their seizures appeared to vary with their menstrual cycles. Nor was I surprised to hear that many women found that their seizures changed at puberty and with menopause. I was concerned to hear women tell me that their menstrual cycles were irregular and to learn from some of my patients about their difficulties in becoming pregnant. There were also stories of miscarriages and complicated pregnancies. Many women (and men) also shared with me concerns about sexuality – problems with

Table 1.1. Special concerns for women with epilepsy

Hormone effects on seizures
Interactions between birth control pills and antiepileptic drugs (AEDs)
Effects of epilepsy on reproductive health
Effects of epilepsy on sexuality
Effects of AEDs on pregnancy and fetal development
Effectiveness and tolerability of AEDs in women

low sexual desire and sexual responsiveness. When I looked at the literature (now more than 10 years ago), I found that many of these issues were not recognized, not well understood, or not considered significant. Some medical writers believed that menstrual-associated seizures did not even exist. Those physicians who did accept the relationship between hormones and seizures sometimes delivered treatments that we now recognize are ineffective, such as hysterectomy and oophorectomy (removal of the uterus and ovaries).

In selecting antiepileptic treatment, I was dismayed to find that most of the information on the effectiveness and tolerability of the medications had been collected almost entirely from men. There was simply not enough information on whether these drugs worked differently in women, had different side effects, or were safe or not safe to use during pregnancy.

Family planning choices for women with epilepsy must take into account the interaction between hormones used for contraception and some antiepileptic drugs (AEDs). Although for more than 10 years some physicians recognized that some AEDs made birth control pills less effective, this information was not widely known by many neurologists and gynecologists. Therefore, some women with epilepsy have experienced unplanned pregnancies despite their best efforts to use contraception correctly.

One of the chief concerns for many women with epilepsy is that seizures and AEDs may make having children more risky. Women with epilepsy have been told that having children was not advisable because of the risks of transmitting epilepsy to a child and of having a baby with major physical or intellectual problems. Women with epilepsy have also been told that their epilepsy makes them unsuitable parents. Until 1982, there were even laws in some states in the USA restricting the ability of people with epilepsy to marry and have children.

Although it has been known for some time that AEDs can cause birth defects, there has been very little information about how these drugs harm the developing fetus and how treatment can be adapted so that there is as little risk as possible. As many new AEDs become available, we have not had the information that allows us to counsel women of childbearing age appropriately regarding the impact of the medications on reproductive health or the medication's safety during pregnancy. This is because, by government policy, women who are capable of becoming pregnant are excluded from the early phases of drug testing when much of the basic information regarding drug dose, effective pharmacokinetics, and tolerability is gathered. Pregnant and lactating (breastfeeding) women are excluded from any exposure to a drug being tested in order to protect the fetus against possible birth defects (teratogenecity). There are over 800 000 women in the USA with epilepsy who are in their childbearing years and probably one-third continue to have seizures despite efforts to achieve control with the older AEDs. That means that new drugs will be used in women during their reproductive years and while pregnant without health-care providers being fully aware of all the potential risks to reproductive health. Government and health-care providers are currently reassessing these drug development policies.

Fortunately, times have changed. A combination of scientific and social advances has brought issues concerning gender differences in medical illnesses to the attention of the general public, government agencies, and the scientific community. It is now recognized that epilepsy is one of the chronic medical conditions that raise special issues for women. This has increased the educational materials available to health-care providers. However, there is still very little literature available for the nonmedical public that comprehensively addresses the biological, psychosocial, and treatment issues faced by women with epilepsy. The Epilepsy Foundation has recognized the importance of encouraging educational outreach as part of the broader based Women with Epilepsy Initiative launched in 1997. This book is a part of that larger effort.

We have been able to assemble national and international experts to address issues of concern for women with epilepsy. Some are scientists researching the causes and consequences of epilepsy, others are health-care providers treating women with epilepsy, and, finally, we hear from women living with epilepsy. We have attempted to be comprehensive and scientifically sound, while interpreting what is sometimes confusing and contradictory scientific information. Each author has selected further materials in each topic for the interested reader. These reference materials are not exhaustive, but have been selected as being particularly important, thorough, and clear. Further information can also be obtained through the National Epilepsy Library at the Epilepsy Foundation or from the Epilepsy Foundation's website at www.epilepsyfoundation.org.

Box 1.1

For more information on the
Women with Epilepsy Initiative
contact the Epilepsy Foundation at
www.epilepsyfoundation.org
1-800-EFA-1000

We have also tried to provide information that will permit a woman with epilepsy to educate herself about optimal medical care – not only for epilepsy, but also to maintain the best general and reproductive health. Epilepsy is best managed when there is a partnership between the patient and health-care provider. Family and friends are also an important part of the team. Ultimately, the woman with epilepsy should understand how to access appropriate services, should know enough about epilepsy to ask the important questions, understand the answers, and be able to anticipate health issues that may arise along the way. The woman who knows most about her disease is in the best situation to benefit from treatment. People with epilepsy can also serve as the most effective advocates to ensure that access to high-quality medical care is maintained, that scientific research continues to address topics of importance to people with epilepsy, and that public misconceptions about epilepsy no longer impede social progress.

2

On being a woman with epilepsy

Lisa Zobian Lindahl

Lisa Lindahl is a member of the Board of Directors of the Epilepsy Foundation, a founder of a successful start-up company (she invented and marketed the first sports bra, the Jogbra), and a woman with epilepsy. Ms Lindahl's efforts were critical to the success of the Epilepsy Foundation's Women with Epilepsy Initiative.

In this chapter, she shares her personal experience and perspective. She discusses what it has been like to live with epilepsy, how she has navigated the medical system, the questions she has asked (and has not always had answered), and how she has become an effective self-advocate. Through Ms Lindahl's voice, you can learn how to be in charge – by getting information, getting noticed, and asking directly for what you need. In Ms Lindahl's thoughtful view, taking responsibility for your own well-being is essential to living well as a woman with epilepsy.

MJM

Epilepsy, as experienced by women, is the subject of this book. Why a whole book? Because so many women, girls, and their families have so many questions, and sometimes it seems there are more questions than answers. This is due, in great part, to the fact that there has only recently been information available about why a woman's experience with epilepsy is different from that of a man's. Further, much of the information was difficult for the average person (like me) to locate. It is hoped that this book will provide the woman with epilepsy with a place to turn for information about those issues that are specific and important to her.

I would like to begin by sharing my own thoughts about and experiences with epilepsy. My credentials for doing so are simply that, having been diagnosed with epilepsy at the age of 3, I have now lived 40-odd years with this disorder. In addition, my volunteer work with the Epilepsy Foundation's

National Office – specifically in our Women and Epilepsy Initiative – has put me in touch with many other women.

As women and as patients, I believe we are dealing with what I refer to as the 'double whammy.' Many women have been culturally conditioned in two ways: (1) the doctor knows best, and (2) men are the authority. Myth or fact, these are two of the assumptions many of us start out with when we embark upon the journey from initial diagnosis to living well with epilepsy. What makes it a double whammy is that most of the neurologists in the USA are male. In addition to my own experiences, I have heard from other women how being a woman *and* having epilepsy can stifle our impetus to speak up when our questions and concerns about how epilepsy impacts our lives are either dismissed or diminished by physicians.

Historically, women have often faced prejudice in what has been a male-dominated health-care system in the USA. In many cases, their symptoms, regardless of the disease, have not been seriously addressed. Women with epilepsy are challenged not only by their epilepsy, but also by the fact that there has been confusion and lack of knowledge in the health-care community about the unique problems facing women with epilepsy.

There are many questions that women or the parents of girls with epilepsy have. These questions can arise early on, with new ones blossoming as we develop and age.

- Will the onset of menses affect the type or severity of my (or my daughter's) seizure disorder?
- How might my reproductive health be affected? Can I have safe pregnancies and healthy babies? Should I breastfeed?
- My experience is that I am far more likely to have seizure activity just prior to menses. Why? Is there anything I can do about it?
- Is the effectiveness of my medication impacted by my monthly hormonal fluctuations? Does medication work the same way on women as it does on men?
- What happens, if anything, as menopause begins and progresses? Are there any interactions between anticonvulsants and the therapies prescribed for menopause, especially hormone replacement therapy (HRT)?

These are just some of the questions facing women who have a seizure disorder. Their primary partner in addressing these issues should be their doctor. Unfortunately, for too many women this partnership has been found wanting. Part of the reason for this is that, until recently, there has been little scientific research into this area.

With a lack of scientific information about the special issues affecting women with epilepsy, guesswork and opinions surface, and they vary. This means that many women with epilepsy have been given misinformation ('You should never have children.') or, if their concerns are acknowledged, they are told there is no information about their unique issues. As a result, we, the patients, are left with many questions unanswered and symptoms ignored.

I am not alone, however. There are a number of women who have the courage to share their experiences:

I began to keep track of the dates of my seizures and found that they occurred prior to my menstruation or during its first two or three days. When I mentioned this to my neurologist, he belittled the possibility of any correlation between the two and stated there were no proven facts to link hormonal cycles and seizures.

The only issue I have regarding my epilepsy has been doctors not taking me seriously when I have told them I thought my seizures and my menstrual cycle were somehow related. It seems to me that when seizures triple in quantity the week before your period and then return to normal afterward, there is something going on.

I was 10 years old when I started menstruating and 30 years old before I got a doctor to take me seriously. I usually got a token pat on the head and the typical 'You're a woman. What do you know?' look. It's a very frustrating and degrading feeling. I hate to see other young girls and teenagers endure what I have to get a doctor to listen.

It is not just learning that researchers are now investigating the links between hormonal changes in women and their seizures that I find important . . . To me, after 43 years of living with seizures, it was great to see women with epilepsy treated as adults with serious questions about treatment, medications, possible causes of their seizures.

The question of catamenial epilepsy has been a long-standing issue for debate within the medical community. Loosely defined, catamenial epilepsy is a term used to describe a seizure disorder that is triggered by hormonal changes during a woman's menstrual cycle. Opinions have varied widely about whether catamenial epilepsy even exists, let alone its cause. The differing opinions on this exist despite the fact that doctors have been hearing women complain and comment upon this phenomenon for over a century.

In fact, women have been reporting the existence of some kind of relationship between hormonal activity and seizure activity since at least the 1800s, when it first appears in medical literature. In 1881, Dr William Gowers reported that about half his female patients seemed to have more seizures before or during their menstrual cycle. Little appears in the literature until 1956, when a paper by J. Laidlaw addressed and described the phenomenon, naming it catamenial epilepsy. No further substantive inquiry was made until over 30 years later. In the last 10 years, this inattention has begun to be remedied. Recently, some medical scientists began to take women's anecdotes seriously and began to do the research.

Every day that goes by, women who are coping with seizure disorders are making decisions and living their lives without adequate information, sometimes with false information and, all too often, with fear. In my files, I have bulging folders filled with letters from women who have suffered from the lack of good information and/or have been confused by differing opinions. Women's lives have been *irrevocably* impacted as a result of being presented with misinformation instead of fact and research results. For instance:

- Upon happily finding out that she was pregnant, one woman was told, (incorrectly) that because of her epilepsy she should have an abortion.
- Another fought to adopt a child because, even though she was a successful biological mother, there was concern about whether she was a 'fit' parent.
- One girl who started having grand mal seizures at puberty was told that they would stop once she had her tonsils and adenoids taken out. She continued to have seizures after the tonsillectomy.
- A young wife in her twenties writes: 'Sexual desire wasn't a problem at first, but over time sex became less desirable because of the pain.' No one ever told her this was related to her epilepsy and to antiepileptic drugs (AEDs).

A chapter from my story

Thankfully, I am one of the lucky ones. Although I experience two different kinds of seizures – one of which is the 'grand mal' convulsion type that is most often associated with the term 'epilepsy' – I have enjoyed long periods of control. Usually, dealing with my seizures has been episodic in nature, a once-a-month concern versus a daily one.

Nonetheless, my own story includes a few disagreeable – and I believe unnecessary – consequences of having a seizure disorder, not the least of which was the virtual loss of more than 2 years of my life. This happened because at one point, in my early thirties, I was so severely over-medicated that I was experiencing daily life in a continual fog. I had many symptoms of chronic depression: tired all the time, unable to think clearly, sad. I had just started my own business and could not afford (in any sense of the word) this obstacle.

Although my memory of this time period is understandably very fuzzy, I can clearly recall that awful sensation of not being able to think, of feeling as though my brain was straining, muffled, clumsy, and slow. Try as I might, I could not shake the murky cloud that seemed to invade my very spirit. The longer I tried, the worse I became, because my failure to 'get better' added to my grief and disappointment in myself.

It took over a year and several doctors, including a psychiatrist, to work out that my problems were, in fact, due to the medicines I was taking, their levels and interactions. It seems the newer drug recently introduced into my treatment plan had a negative, slowly cumulative interaction with my other prescribed AED. The result was an ever-increasing depressant effect. Imagine my tremendous relief to discover that this oppressive fog was not really *me*. I was not weak; I was not emotionally troubled. *I was not crazy!* I was just experiencing medication side effects.

The medication was adjusted, well below the 'recommended therapeutic level' (a level that had been established by tests done primarily on men), and I started to get well. It took months before I really felt like myself again. Then, once I was well, I got angry. Why had everyone been so quick to assume that my complaints were emotionally based rather than physically or chemically induced? Having not been forewarned about such a possibility, I had spent far too long, initially, thinking that 'This fog is all in my imagination; get over it.'

It became clear to me that my epilepsy, improperly managed, would have a devastating impact on my life and livelihood if I did not take charge of my health. I was living alone – a new circumstance and daunting enough in itself – and 'taking care of myself' could no longer just entail taking the prescribed pills. I could no longer relinquish the final responsibility for decisions regarding my care to the doctor. Rather, the doctor was an expert consultant to me and I was responsible for my own care and finally in control.

It sounds ridiculously self-evident, doesn't it? But it wasn't for me, and it isn't for many other women who – even in the face of their own contradicting perceptions – trust that 'Doctor knows best.'

When a woman *does* learn to express her opinion or talk about her experiences, she still may not be taken seriously. As evidenced by the quotes at the beginning of this chapter as well as by my own experience, our perceptions have at times been trivialized. A woman's knowledge about her seizures may not be validated and so many women may decide that 'the doctor knows best:' 'The doctor is right, therefore I am wrong.' But if we later discover that the doctor was wrong, we may feel anger, disbelief, and even betrayal. When we come to terms with the fact that, as the patient or the 'consumer' of the medical care, we are the ones who reap the benefit and/or pay the price of medical decisions, then we must take ultimate responsibility.

With this realization, I began to question everything. I became a very 'discriminating' patient and some of the doctors I dealt with were uncomfortable about what they perceived as my skepticism. I persisted until I found those with whom I could work. Fortunately, this has become a great deal easier in the last few years as more doctors recognize the value of their patients' perspective and are willing to work in partnership with her.

When I began to take charge of my condition, I realized that my seizures were hormone sensitive and, although I did not know the name then, I am aware now that I have catamenial epilepsy. Intitially, according to the doctors I first consulted, I did not. The first grand mal convulsion (generalized tonic–clonic seizure) I had was at the onset of menses at the age of 12. This was the first indication of a relationship between my seizures and my hormones. Now, over 35 years later, I can look back and clearly view this on-going phenomenon. I have years of charts and calendars. Its predictability was so great that I was able to plan business travel and other obligations around what I came to know as my 'high-risk' time – the week just prior to my period.

This very predictability was one of the reasons that I consider myself 'lucky.' It made having a seizure disorder somewhat more manageable. Those happy days are gone. Now peri-menopausal, my seizure pattern is no longer predictable. I believe this is due to my hormonal fluctuations during this time of change. Without the ability to predict high-risk times, I must devise different methods to manage my disorder.

It was only 7 years ago that I learned that there was scientific research going on around the issue of catamenial epilepsy. For me, it was a red-letter day when I saw a doctor get up and explain, very simply on a flip chart with a little diagram, how and why hormones can trigger seizure activity.

Taking charge: one woman's approach to seizure management

To be in charge of one's seizure disorder one must practice seizure management. *I* must manage the disorder; the disorder must not manage me. Just as I am responsible for work, a household, or budget management, I am also responsible for the management of the control of my epilepsy. Beyond listening to your own body's messages, part of being responsible is to become educated about your particular seizure type and keep up with advances in therapies.

However, successful seizure management is not confined to medical considerations. Beyond managing your seizure disorder in terms of your AEDs and their levels, there are all the ways to manage it that have to do with lifestyle choices – daily living and working patterns and habits.

My life as a busy and successful entrepreneur, a single woman living alone, confronted and defied many of the obstacles associated with living with epilepsy.

For example, early morning is always a risky time for me because my seizures, if they are going to appear, seem to do so at that time of day. I had been told that this was in response to any degree of sleep deprivation and/or a change in sleep patterns. As a result, I tried never to schedule any early-morning business meetings and I would work at home until I knew I was going to be all right. If someone else set an early meeting, I always let it be known that I would do my best, but could not guarantee my attendance – especially if it was during a pre-menstrual week. Further, if I had to travel, I would fly the night before rather than early on the morning of the meeting. The hotel room expense was worth the peace of mind and extra sleep (see Table 2.1 for tips on managing your seizures).

Recognizing the choices that you have, asking yourself questions like those listed in Table 2.1, and formulating their solutions can put you in more control

Table 2.1. Managing your seizures

Have you tracked your seizure activity on a calendar to identify any patterns and improve your ability to predict high-risk times?

Are you aware of any factors that have helped to trigger seizures in the past, such as lack of sleep, stress, hormonal cycles, flashing lights, etc.?

Are there certain times of day that you are most likely to have seizures?

Is your home on a public transportation route? If not, is it serviced by a cab company?

Have you told coworkers about your epilepsy? If not, what are the considerations that are holding you back from sharing this information? Does it serve you best to tell them or not tell them?

Do those consistently around you know how to recognize and respond appropriately to a seizure?

Is there someone in your life you can count on for help and 'back-up' at those times that you need it? If not, how might you find someone?

For travel, do you have some kind of access to 24-hour emergency medical care? (I have a credit card that offers such assistance all over the world. This has greatly appeased my anxiety about, among other more dramatic possibilities, ever losing my pills while away from home and my local pharmacy.)

---

of your epilepsy. I have found the quote: 'God grant me the courage to change the things I can, the serenity to accept those I cannot, and the wisdom to know the difference' a helpful tool to focus on what is really important.

The fear factor

Although no one likes to acknowledge that they are afraid, when first diagnosed, epilepsy can seem frightening. But it is vital to your long-term well-being that you confront your fears sooner, rather than later. In my experience, it has been rare that any epilepsy-related fears are talked about, but it is important to address them openly.

Everyone who takes medication for epilepsy has concerns about possible side effects. For me, the fear of cognitive impairment has always loomed large. Hair loss, hypertrophy of the gums, weight gain, excessive facial hair – these are some others. With the strong emphasis our society places on a woman's physical appearance, just the threat of these side effects can be a concern.

Besides the visible side effects of various AEDs, there are two other areas in which women may have epilepsy-related fears. The first is child-bearing and raising. Most women with epilepsy have successfully borne and raised their children. But these data do not always relieve the anxiety that some women with epilepsy may feel. When you are worried about your own safety, it can be difficult to imagine being responsible for an infant as well.

The second area of concern is that of physical safety, especially the risk of sexual assault during, or just after, a seizure. The temporary loss of awareness with some seizures and confusion after them can make a woman feel vulnerable. Although such incidents are not believed to be numerous, victimization is an understandable apprehension.

At different times in my life different fears have dominated. As a little girl on phenytoin, I was afraid my eyebrows would grow together over my nose (they didn't). As a young woman, I was worried that if I had a child I would be unable to breastfeed. As a business owner and 'frequent flyer', I was afraid that I would have a seizure in some unknown place and be at the mercy of strangers. (In fact, I have had seizures in such places. In each incident, far from being in danger, the aforementioned 'strangers' took good and gentle care of me.) Now, as a middle-aged woman, I am concerned about the effect of menopause on epilepsy. While I do not dwell on my fears, ignoring them only leads to denial, which can cause carelessness and mismanagement of my epilepsy. With successful seizure management I can diminish the impact of epilepsy-related fear in my life.

In reality, it is not possible to discuss all of the fears that women with epilepsy might encounter. It is a complex and sensitive subject. The reaction to epilepsy is unique to each individual, much as a seizure disorder itself manifests uniquely in each person. I touch on it here not to introduce, promote or further fear, but to demonstrate that none of us is alone in the apprehensions we may feel.

Looking forward

A few years ago, the National Health Council stated in their report *Trends in Women's Health Care*:

In the next decade women's health advocates will see...an explosion of biomedical and behavioral information defining gender differences in areas ranging from drug absorption rates to patterns of diagnostic bias and gender-specific treatments....Most importantly, hormonal research will guide medicine into new territory.

It is even more important, however, that any such 'new territory' offers some new solutions to the very old problems facing women with epilepsy today. It is my hope that, with the research being done today, our grand-daughters' generation will have better answers and be better equipped to deal with epilepsy.

The epilepsy community – both professionals and patients – has become far more aware of the unique issues that face women with epilepsy. Although there is still a long way to go, it is time to move away from the indictment of past neglect to excitement about the future possibilities – even for a cure. A girl or woman who is diagnosed with epilepsy today has a brighter outlook. The relationship between a woman's biology and her seizure disorder represents a whole new frontier for epilepsy research. For the patient, having information and acquiring greater understanding create a feeling of control and empowerment. This by itself can increase significantly the quality of life of the patient – no matter how severe her epilepsy.

However, to seek solutions for women with epilepsy and their unique problems is, I believe, more than a little dependent upon us, the very women affected. *We must make our voices heard.* We must become educated and stay educated, so that we can monitor our own care. We must question, to understand better. We must learn to manage the seizure disorder as we manage other responsibilities and not be ruled by our fears. Most importantly, we must trust what our own bodies are telling us.

3

The woman with epilepsy: a historical perspective

Orrin Devinsky

Dr Orrin Devinsky is an eminent epilepsy specialist and former member of the Professional Advisory Board of the Epilepsy Foundation. In this chapter, he reviews the medical history of epilepsy as it relates to women, drawing on his own extensive knowledge about epilepsy, its treatment, and an impressive personal collection of historical texts. Where we are now relates to where we have been. The medical and social histories of epilepsy are filled with stories of wrong information and wrong action. Much of the misunderstanding has impacted women especially. They were thought to suffer from gynecological diseases, unhealthy sexual impulses, and were even considered to be witches. Modern-day therapies have improved the life of the woman with epilepsy. Advances in medical knowledge have put old superstitions and fears to rest. Yet stigma persists. The best way to address this stigma is to understand the source and have access to the information that will end discrimination.

MJM

Epilepsy has affected humans since the dawn of the species and has been recognized since the earliest medical writings. Few medical conditions have attracted so much attention and controversy. Throughout history, people with epilepsy, as well as their families, suffered unfairly because of the ignorance of others. Fortunately, the stigma and fear generated by the words seizure and epilepsy have increasingly diminished during the last century, and the majority of those with seizure disorders now lead a normal life.

The earliest medical texts on epilepsy were on Egyptian papyri and Babylonian cuneiform tablets. The Babylonians (circa 1067–1046 BC) believed that epilepsy was caused by demons and ghosts who controlled some individuals (Wilson-Kinnier and Reynolds, 1990).

The Greek physician Hippocrates wrote the first book on epilepsy, *On the Sacred Disease*, around 400 BC. He recognized that epilepsy was a brain dysfunction and argued against the ideas that seizures were a curse from the gods and that people with epilepsy could predict the future.

Hippocrates wrote:

I am about to discuss the disease called 'sacred.' It is not in my opinion any more divine or more sacred than other diseases, but has a natural cause, and its supposed divine origin is due to men's inexperience, and to their wonder at its peculiar character. Now while men continue to believe in its divine origin because they are at a loss to understand it, they really disprove its divinity by the facile method of healing which they adopt, consisting as it does of purifications and incantations. But if it is to be considered divine just because it is wonderful, there would be not one sacred disease but many.

However, even Hippocrates' authority could not remove the superstition and intense stigma surrounding epilepsy. For centuries, epilepsy was considered a curse of the gods, or worse. The idea that epilepsy was an evil possession led to social isolation for the one who had epilepsy and, in many cases, for his or her family as well.

On seeing a person with epilepsy, medical authorities after Hippocrates often recommended spitting to 'throw back' the contagion (Pliny, 1856–65). Romans sent away family members with epilepsy, to avoid 'contamination' (Apuleius, 1914). Even slaves shunned other slaves with epilepsy; they spat at them and avoided sharing their food or drink.

To most ancients, epilepsy was a horrid affliction. References throughout ancient Greek and Roman medical texts indicate that the person with epilepsy was viewed with disgust, and that the connotations of 'sacred' may have largely reflected the frightening, awesome, and taboo aspects of the disorder. The seizure of a person's soul and body by gods or demons may have simultaneously made epilepsy sacred and untouchable (Temkin, 1971).

Those with popular and religious beliefs in the supernatural and demonic side of epilepsy outnumbered the minority that looked for nonsupernatural causation.

Possession, magic, and witchcraft became dominant themes applied to epilepsy and its origins during the Middle Ages; diagnosing and treating possession were the focal points of epilepsy care. The handbook on witch-hunting *Malleus Maleficarum*, written by two Dominican friars under papal authority in 1494, identified witches by the presence of certain characteristics, including seizures. The book also said that witches could cause epilepsy to develop: 'For although greater difficulty may be felt in believing that witches are able to cause leprosy or epilepsy, since these diseases generally arise from some long-standing physical predisposition or defect, none the less it has sometimes been found that even these have been caused by witchcraft' (Institoris, 1928, p. 136). The *Malleus* brought a wave of persecution and torture, and led to an estimated 100 000 to 1 000 000 women being put to death.

Throughout the Middle Ages, some physicians (e.g., Hieronymus Gabucinius, Johann Weyer, Levinus Lemnius) upheld the Hippocratic wisdom, asserting that epilepsy was a natural disorder. However, it was believed to be infectious, as were bubonic plague, tuberculosis, scabies, Erysiphales, anthrax, trachoma, and leprosy (Lennox and Lennox, 1960).

During the eighteenth century's Enlightenment, the Hippocratic belief – epilepsy as a physical disorder of the brain, not a supernatural curse – gained acceptance. During the same time, interest in the role of the moon as a cause of epilepsy and insanity (lunacy is from the word *luna*, meaning moon) had wider acceptance, as did the role of masturbation. The use of amulets, rings, charms, holy rituals, incantations, human skull bones, and magical therapies waned during the eighteenth century.

In the early nineteenth century, the first asylums were created to house psychiatric and epileptic patients. The fear that epilepsy was contagious was 'confirmed,' probably through the presentation of nonepileptic psychogenic seizures in the psychiatric population, leading to a separation of these two groups. For example, the French psychiatrist Esquirol (1845) noted that he feared the spread of epilepsy to those who only had mental disorders. Asylums provided the first opportunity for the study and systematic observation of epilepsy in various populations. The segregation of the two populations also led to the creation of hospitals for the paralyzed and epileptic in the late 1800s – from Queen Square in London (1860) to Blackwell's Island in New York (1867). In the early nineteenth century, epilepsy colonies were established in many states, such as the Craig Colony in Sonyea, New York. These epilepsy colonies segregated women and men (Fig. 3.1).

Before the twentieth century, epilepsy meant convulsive attacks, i.e., tonic–clonic seizures (grand mal seizures, convulsions). Thus, throughout much of recorded history, children and adults with absence seizures and simple and complex partial seizures were never diagnosed and treated for epilepsy. This

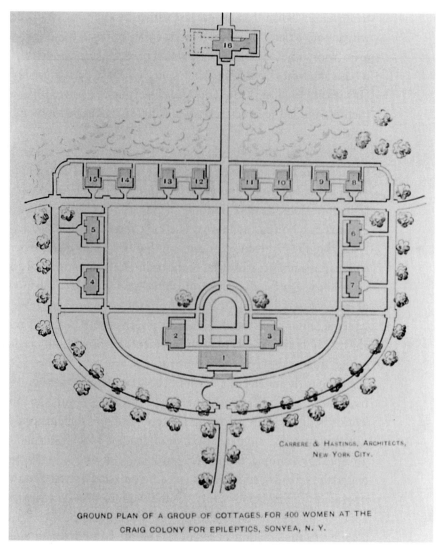

GROUND PLAN OF A GROUP OF COTTAGES FOR 400 WOMEN AT THE
CRAIG COLONY FOR EPILEPTICS, SONYEA, N. Y.

Figure 3.1   Plans for cottages for 400 women at the Craig Colony for Epileptics in Sonyea, NY.

group probably comprised about half of those with epilepsy. Furthermore, many with tonic–clonic seizures mainly had absence or complex partial seizures, and the convulsions may well have occurred during sleep or in the privacy of their home, allowing concealment of the disorder. The failure to recognize the nonconvulsive forms of epileptic seizures and the ability to conceal the convulsive forms were largely a blessing, because effective treatments were lacking and stigma was more intense and more pervasive.

At the turn of the twentieth century, epilepsy 'colonies' were the state-of-the-art 'progressive' care for those with epilepsy. These colonies offered rest, bromides and systematic study, and a way for wealthy families to rid themselves of the embarrassment and discomfort of epilepsy. Even in 1925, James Leuba's classic monograph on religious mysticism said: 'Among the dread diseases that afflict humanity there is only one that interests us quite particularly; that disease is epilepsy.'

In the mid-twentieth century in the USA, epilepsy was viewed as a social as well as a medical disease. Individuals were isolated and legislated against in employment and in laws regarding driving, marrying, reproducing, and becoming a parent. Families hid the presence of epilepsy, fearing stigma against themselves and limited marriage opportunities for relatives.

Epilepsy in women: a history

Two surveys of the history of epilepsy (Lennox and Lennox, 1960; Temkin, 1971) show a strong male bias in the medical writings on the diagnosis, causation, and treatment of people with epilepsy from ancient to more recent times. Medical writings on epilepsy (and other disorders) from ancient Semites, Greeks, Romans, and through the Middle Ages, Renaissance, and Enlightenment have focused on males with the disorder. The notable exceptions concern witchcraft and hysteria. Hysteria is now referred to as conversion disorder, in which a person develops symptoms that suggest a neurological or medical disorder but the symptoms result from psychological factors.

The history of hysteria is strongly tied to epilepsy. Egyptian papyri discuss disturbances resulting from movement of the womb. The Hippocratic writings gave this the name *hysteria* (from womb, *hystera*). Initially, Greek writings often referred to hysteria in connection with respiratory difficulties. The writings said that women deprived of sexual relations developed a dry, atrophic uterus that would rise in the body to find moisture, thus impeding breathing. When the womb came to rest in the abdomen, it caused epilepsy (Hippocrates; Veith, 1965). During the time of Hippocrates, convulsions in women were believed to result from either hysteria or epilepsy. Differential diagnosis, essential for appropriate therapy, was sometimes accomplished by digital pressure on the woman's abdomen. If the pressure was felt, the disorder was hysteria; if not, it was probably epilepsy. (Hippocrates; Veith, 1965). Later, Greeks believed that hysterical loss of consciousness due to upward migration of the womb was not accompanied by convulsive movements. Paracelsus, in the early sixteenth century, observed that if the womb 'touches the heart the convulsion is similar to epilepsy with all its symptoms.'

The modern history of hysteria and epilepsy began with Willis, who, in 1684, first suggested that hysteria was a disorder of brain function and emphasized the association of epilepsy and hysteria, speculating that both disorders share a similar mechanism (Veith, 1965). However, the coexistence of hysteria (conversion disorder) and epilepsy within one patient was first recognized in 1836 by Beau. Shortly after this, Esquirol (1845) observed 'hysteric patients who are at the same time epileptics . . . With a little practice one could recognize very well, when the attacks are separate, to which of the two diseases the convulsions belong to which the patient is actually prey.' Around the same time, Landouzy (1846) postulated 'the coexistence of two neuroses, with distinct attacks,' to which he gave the name 'hystero-epilepsy with separate crises.' Subsequently, the coexistence of the two disorders was discussed by Trousseau (1868), Dostoyevsky (1881), D'Olier (1882), and Gowers (1888), with attention focused on differentiating the two types of seizures. Perhaps the greatest contribution was made by Charcot, who described four patterns of coexistent hysteria and epilepsy: (1) hysteria supervening in a patient already epileptic, (2) epilepsy supervening in a patient already hysteric, (3) convulsive hysteria coexisting with epileptic vertigo, and (4) epilepsy developing upon the results of hysteria, nonconvulsive (e.g., contracture, anesthesia) (quoted by D'Olier, 1882).

The modern era of psychiatry was partly ushered in by Mesmerism (Fig. 3.2), and laid the foundation for hypnosis and the more rigorous late nineteenth century study of hysteria. As Figure 3.2 shows, a large portion of Dr Mesmer's clients were women. The study of hysteria was later advanced by Charcot and colleagues at the Salpetriere in Paris, where studies on hysteria and hysteroepilepsy flourished (Figs. 3.3 and 3.4).

The ancient Greek diagnostic maneuver of abdominal compression evolved in nineteenth century France to ovarian compression (believed to induce hysterical convulsion) or prolonged pressure (to arrrest hysterical seizure).

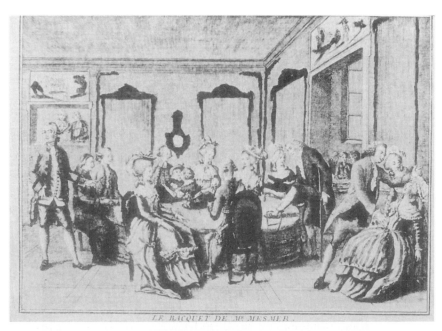

Figure 3.2   A treatment session by Dr Mesmer. (From the collection of Dr J.M. published in *Nouvelle Iconographie De Salpætriére,* late nineteenth century.)

Gowers reported the effectiveness of French neurologist Jean-Martin Charcot's ovarian compression in the classic *A Manual of Diseases of the Nervous System* (1888): 'Pressure on the tender ovarian region, or other tender hysterogenic spots, as already stated, sometimes induces an attack, and prolonged pressure will often arrest the seizure. Sometimes the ovarian compression simply arrests the coordinate movements, and causes tonic spasm.' Yet, in Gowers' earlier first edition of *Epilepsy and Other Chronic Convulsive Disorders* in 1881, he made the following comments: 'Ovarian compression, which is so effective in inducing and in cutting short the attacks of hystero-epilepsy at the Salpetriere Hospital often as already stated, fails to produce a marked effect in patients in this country, although ovarian tenderness is by no means uncommon.'

The role of menstruation

Menarche, menstruation, and menopause have been associated with changes in epileptic seizure activity for centuries. The Hippocratic writings noted

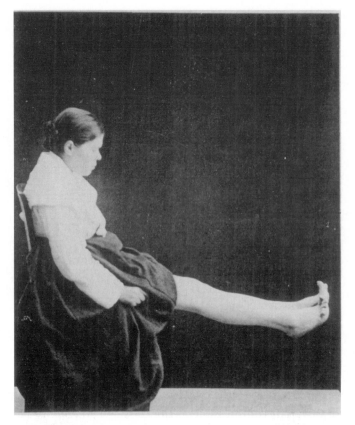

Figure 3.3   A patient with hysteria. (Published in *Nouvelle Iconographie De Salpætriére*, 1890.)

that cessation of the menstrual flux could cause epileptic seizures. Galen of Pergamon opined that regular menses helped prevent epilepsy (Temkin, 1971). Bernard of Gordon, in 1542, stated that seizures associated with menstruation were not curable (Temkin, 1971).

In the first major American textbook on epilepsy, M. Gonzalez Echeverria (1870) provided this commentary:

The commencement and the arrest of menstruation range conspicuously among the organic changes inducing epilepsy. The intervention of these causes appears more efficient than any other acting on the female sex. It is a trite remark that once fairly established epilepsy produces irregularities of the catamenia [menstruation]. I find in looking over the period of this complication in individual cases that, the younger the female the earlier the trouble existed, it being seldom delayed beyond the fourth month of the

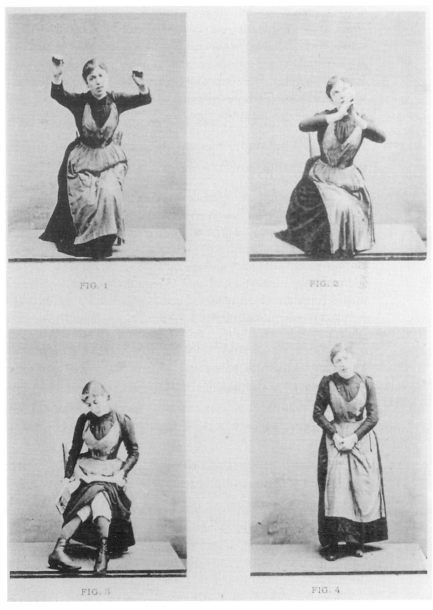

Figure 3.4   A patient with hysteria. (Published in *Nouvelle Iconographie De Salpætriére*, 1890.)

active progress of spasms; whereas in those females affected after puberty, or at more advanced age, the mischief was not so particularly noticeable and obvious only in the severer cases . . . I fail to trace any noxious association, or more frequent development, of the epileptic attacks with the age of menopause . . . In all the forms of epilepsy dating from infancy, the establishment of menstruation was more or less delayed, the paroxysms having usually increased in severity on or about the menstrual period; and in one instance menstruation never took place. (pp. 212–13).

Echeverria had more observations on the causes and provocative factors of epilepsy among women:

There is one circumstance connected with the establishment of puberty which forms the dominant feature of this age, namely, the sexual orgasm. This secretly brooded fever is as peculiar to the human as to other animal species. When undisturbed in its operation, our organic frame assumes its procreative power . . . but if held in restraint . . . then all kinds of nervous disorders hand over the path marked out to the youth . . . to feebleness and depression . . . (they) display themselves with more vivid and distressing forms in woman, condemned by social life to a position which draws after it her greater weakness to stand the sexual instinct. (1870, p. 214)

Echevarria also quoted the leading British psychiatrist of the time, Henry Maudsley, who considered feelings of sexual passion a factor in causing insanity in women: ' . . . its influence on every pulse of organic life, revolutionizing the entire nature, conscious and unconscious . . . when there is no vicarious outlet for its energy . . . restlessness and irritability . . . instinctive frenzy' (Maudsley, 1867, p. 202).

Thus, added Echeverria (1870, p. 215), 'it is not, therefore, difficult to understand how unnatural attempts to menstruation – first evidence of puberty – may superinduce the actual appearances of epilepsy in a constitution so much disturbed and irritable.' He then noted the clear relation, in many women, between an exacerbation of epileptic attacks and uterine functions, specifically 'from unhealthy excitement by the established uterine discharge.'

Echeverria (1881) moved beyond uterine position and explored the neglected role of the ovaries:

Ovarian derangement accompanies uterine disease generally, and perseveres as the main source of trouble in these cases. We overlooked the ovaries, carrying our sight not much beyond the cervical canal exposed by the speculum. There is a growing reaction against the consequent surgical interference that has prevailed to this day in uterine therapeutics ... amenorrhea, dysmenorrhea, and other nervous disorders exhibited by females ... some unknown morbid state of the ovaries.

Bouchet and Cazauvieilh (1825) provided the first statistics, albeit indirect, on catamenial epilepsy. In 3 of 14 women with epilepsy, difficult menstruation was considered a causative factor. Gowers recorded a 39% prevalence of catamenial seizures in 82 women with epilepsy. In the second edition of his classic monograph on epilepsy, Gowers (1901) provided an update: 'In one twelfth no attacks occurred at the time of menstruation; in one third there was no difference at these times; in more than half the attacks were worse at the monthly periods. Most frequently they were worse before the period; next in frequency during the period, and much less frequently after the period.'

Spratling's 1904 monograph on epilepsy stated that, in patients with dysmenorrhea, the ovaries are often enlarged and cystic, and their removal often lessens the frequency and severity of the seizures. This is one form of the 'menstrual epilepsies.' However, when the ovaries are normal and the epileptic seizures are more frequent at the menstrual period, they should not be removed: 'Make careful inquiry into the possible influence of perverted functions on the part of the reproductive organs in any case of epilepsy among women occurring after puberty and before the menopause.' Spratling later gave other guidelines for removal of the ovaries in women with epilepsy. They should be removed if (1) attacks begin around puberty; (2) attacks occur in close conjunction with the menstrual cycle; (3) no hereditary cause of epilepsy is found; and (4) after years of epilepsy, the functioning of the mind is not appreciably impaired.

Marriage and pregnancy

A change in epilepsy with pregnancy was recognized in the late 1500s and the 1600s, (Fernelius, 1577; Schenckius, 1644), with additional cases described by La Motte and Tissot in the 1700s. In most instances, women with epilepsy had an increase in convulsions during pregnancy, although in some cases seizures abated during pregnancy, and rarely began during pregnancy. (Sieveking observed that one woman had onset of epilepsy during pregnancy.) La Motte (1771) described an unusual case: a woman, who had been pregnant eight times, only suffered convulsions after she conceived a male child.

Legal barriers to marriage for men and women with epilepsy represent a black page in the history of epilepsy in the USA. These laws persisted in some states into the mid-nineteenth century. In the early nineteenth century, marriage was recommended, mainly for women with epilepsy, as a method to improve epilepsy. For example, Prichard (1822) described a woman with catamenial epilepsy for 4 years. When she married and became pregnant, seizures ceased. Prichard believed that marriage could improve catamenial seizures, even if a woman did not become pregnant.

In 1881, Echeverria provided the first medical paper summarizing medical, popular, and legal opinions on marriage and epilepsy. In 1901, Gowers related his observations, dispelling the ancient views that sexual abstinence provoked seizures while sexual activity could stop them: 'Attacks which have resisted treatment before marriage usually persist afterwards without any considerable change. There is no evidence to show that marital relations, in moderation, have any influence on the disease.' Gowers (1901, p. 305) offers a thoughtful and sensitive discussion of issues related to the hereditary nature of some epilepsies and how this affects the medical recommendations toward marriage and conception:

> Whenever evidence of inheritance can be discerned, the danger of transmission is definite, and cannot be ignored. The amount of risk is roughly proportioned to the extent of traceable antecedent disease. Exceptions are frequent in the relation between the two . . . As in all questions of probability, the rules which are true of a number taken together, often fail in individual instances. No precise forecast can therefore ever be given . . . For the welfare of the community . . . members of families with clear inheritance abstained from the risk of transmitting disease . . . But there is a large class of cases in which it is very difficult to give an opinion . . . cases in which the disease has all the features of idiopathic epilepsy . . . but no inheritance can be traced.

Gowers goes on to describe the despair of parents with seizures or mental disorders who have children with similar afflictions, which, he notes, may skip a generation.

The view of epilepsy experts in the USA shortly after the turn of the twentieth century was somewhat less sympathetic. Spratling's (1904) landmark monograph on epilepsy, based on his experience with outpatients and his role as the medical superintendent of the Craig Colony for Epileptics (the first major colony in the USA, located in upstate New York), offers a pessimistic view on epilepsy and marriage:

The marriage of epileptics is sometimes urged for its supposed favorable influence on the disease, but so far as my observation goes . . . (marriage has) no beneficial effect on the disease. Irrespective of this, marriage confers a license for the creation of a diseased progeny generally lower in mental, moral, and physical stamina than their antecedents. This fact alone should be sufficient to deny the epileptic the right of marriage in fully ninety-five out of every hundred cases in which it is sought (p. 302–3).

In the first edition of the most popular American text on neurology in the first half of the twentieth century, Munson (1913) provided a sobering social view of epilepsy: 'Institutional treatment for all epileptics is advocated as far as the public purse will permit . . . prophylaxis by legal means as far as possible – segregation, operation, limitation of marriage; but above all by the education of the public to the dangers of mating between the unfit.' On limiting marriage among persons with epilepsy, Munson said, 'Legal limitation of marriage . . . is not . . . sufficiently far-reaching, as many of the most dangerous matings (from the eugenics standpoint) are consummated outside the bonds of wedlock. A few States have enacted such laws, but they are at present more or less inoperative, on account of the lack of a sentiment in their favor' (p. 271).

The effects of maternal convulsions and the potential hazards of medical therapy on the fetus were recognized in the nineteenth century. Although some argued that maternal convulsions did not affect the developing fetus (Laforgue, 1867), Echeverria cared for four women who had convulsions throughout pregnancy and gave birth to children who died in convulsions shortly after birth. Another woman he cared for had a series of convulsions and miscarried 2 days after the last attack. However, he also recorded two women treated with bromides throughout pregnancy who gave birth to healthy babies.

Gowers' (1901) experience was that most women enjoyed a reduction in seizure frequency during pregnancy, and that most of the others had no change in seizure frequency. He also noted that childbirth is rarely complicated by seizures and, if a seizure occurs during labor, it 'has not usually any unfavourable effect.'

Therapies for epilepsy

Historically, therapies prescribed for epilepsy have been extremely varied, and limited only by imagination, but not necessarily pain tolerance or efficacy. Edward Sieveking, the English neurologist, observed, 'There is scarcely a substance in the world capable of passing through the gullet of man that has not at one time or another enjoyed the reputation of being an antiepileptic.' Swallowed remedies included cups of blood from recently dead humans, powdered human skull, mistletoe, digitalis, silver nitrate, zinc oxide, and vulture liver (Temkin, 1971; Scott, 1993). Other therapies included bloodletting, purging, vomiting, diuresis, sweating, recommendation for increased coital activity or abstinence, pressing a hot metal button or iron on the head to drain a pernicious humor, or trephining (opening) the skull to allow evil spirits to escape.

Bromides were the first effective therapy for epileptic seizures. In 1857, Charles Locock, a society doctor and obstetrician to Queen Victoria, noted that bromides were effective in a group of females with hystero-epilepsy. The rationale for the therapy was never stated by Locock, but was probably related indirectly to onanism (masturbation). Onanism had long been considered a cause of epilepsy as well as of madness. Even Gowers, in 1881, noted:

It was very difficult to determine the influence of masturbation as a cause of epilepsy. The habit is common in epileptic boys, as in others, but we cannot infer that, in all such cases, it is the cause of the disease. The etiological relation can only be regarded as established when the arrest of the habit, as by circumcision, arrests the disease. But the converse is not true; the continuance of the disease after the arrest of the practice does not disprove the relationship, because, when the 'convulsive habit' is established, it frequently persists after its cause has ceased to be effective (p. 25).

In 1850, Georges Huette reported the effectiveness of bromides in causing impotence in men and effectively treating vivid imagination and masturbation. Based on these results, Locock began to use bromides for hysteria in young women. With some success in this disorder, he extended the bromide therapy to 'hysterical epilepsy' when the epileptic attacks 'only occurred during the catamenial period, except under otherwise strong exciting causes' (Temkin, 1971, p. 298). Seizures were cured in 13 of 14 of these cases (Sieveking, 1861, p. 528). Reynolds, in his monograph on epilepsy written 4 years after Locock's report, did not share his successful responses. Wilks, who doubted Locock's theory of bromides acting on ovarian irritation, reported his successful therapy of men and women with epilepsy in 1861.

J. Russell Reynolds, an English neurologist, made the following observation regarding bromides in his great monograph on epilepsy (1861, pp. 332–3):

Bromide of potassium was strongly recommended by Sir Charles Locock in those cases of epilepsy where the attacks recurred only at the menstrual periods. Such cases are not of frequent occurrence; although it is common enough to meet with women whose fits are more numerous during or just before the catamenial discharge. In the latter class I have tried bromide of potassium, and carried it on until the menses have ceased, but have witnessed no diminution of the attacks. There is evidence to show that this medicine will distinctly diminish erotic tendencies in some cases, and especially in the female sex; whereas there are other cases in which it as distinctly fails...It has appeared to be of much use in some cases of hysteria.

Similarly, concerning bromides, Sieveking wrote: 'though I have not enjoyed the same amount of success I have found it decidedly beneficial. In one case where the irritation of sexual apparatus was very marked a permanent cure seemed to be attributable to it.'

William Alexander's 1889 text, *The Treatment of Epilepsy*, provides some of the clearest descriptions of therapies directed specifically at women. He noted that masturbation was often a result – not a cause – of epilepsy in males. In a personal series of four castrations in males, he noted no improvement of epilepsy, although he reported other physicians who did find this procedure beneficial. About women, he said:

In women, the menstrual functions are credited with great potency in producing epilepsy. I have never performed oophorectomy [surgical removal of the ovaries] for epilepsy, but Mr. Lawson Tait has operated on several cases, and speaks of them rather favourably in his book on 'Diseases of the Ovaries.' Some time afterwards, in conversation with me, he expressed his disappointment at the ultimate results, the disease recurring after a longer or shorter time in the majority of cases... These operations, to be useful, should be performed at once, when epilepsy occurs; but the disease is of so uncertain character, that it would only be in very rare cases that either surgeon or patient would submit to an operation that would, in the female, be attended with some amount of risk, and that in both sexes would deprive them of what every one prizes so much, the capability of procreation (p. 121).

Alexander performed a ligature of the vertebral arteries on one woman with epilepsy. The procedure had no effect on her epilepsy. Because her 'fits' began when she had menstrual derangement, he examined her uterine organs and found a retroversion of the uterus. He shortened the round ligaments, bringing the uterus back to its normal position, and she subsequently had two children and 6 years of seizure freedom when he reported her case. Another woman treated in a similar manner continued to have epileptic attacks despite being 'stupefied with bromide' so that he could 'not rely upon her for answers.'

Clitoridectomy was used during the late nineteenth century for treating women with epilepsy, as was castration for some men (Duffy, 1963).

Therapy for people with epilepsy has advanced dramatically from early 1900s when the toxic bromides and phenobarbital were often increased to extinguish seizures at the cost of vanquishing the person's mind and debilitating their body. The pace of progress has varied, with rapid advances in one area accompanied by stagnation in others. During the twentieth century, women with epilepsy have benefited from greater understanding of epilepsy, major advances in diagnostic tools, awareness, and attempts to formulate individualized, safe approaches to special issues such as birth control, pregnancy, sexual function, and menopause.

Summary

It is easy to look back on the past with a condescending modern eye, viewing a primitive and barbaric landscape of medical care. This is unfair and inaccurate. The physicians, scientists, families, and patients were intricately tied to the fabric of their society and beliefs. So are we. The eugenics movement and the recommendation that people with epilepsy be prevented from reproduction were considered progressive, integrating principles of natural selection into human advancement. A new and largely correct theory was adapted to the social–medical entity of epilepsy with recommendations we now view as horrific. Will the two-class system of medical care in many parts of our country appear any less barbaric to future generations? There are many areas where our understanding and therapies are sorely lacking. Greater cooperation between patient and doctor will help provide some of these answers.

SELECTED REFERENCES

Alexander W. *The Treatment of Epilepsy*. Pentland, Edinburgh, 1889.

Apuleius. *Apulei apologia*. Introduction and commentary by Butler HE, Owen AS. Clarendon Press, Oxford, 1914.

Beau B. Recherches statisques pour servir a l'histoire de l'epilepsie et de l'hysterie. *Arch Gen Med*, 2e serie 1836; 11:328–52.

Bouchet C, Cazauvieilh D. De l'epilepsie considere dans ses rapports avec l'alienation mentale. *Arch Gen Med* 1825; 9:510–42.

D'Olier M. On the coexistence of hysteria and epilepsy, with distinct manifestations of two neuroses. *Alienist Neurologist* 1882; 3:178–93.

Dostoyevsky F. *The Brothers Karamzov*. Transl. Magarshack D. Penguin, Hammondsworth, 1881.

Duffy J. Masturbation and clitoridectomy: a nineteenth century view. *JAMA* 1963; 186:246–8.

Echeverria MG. *On Epilepsy: Anatomo-Pathological and Clinical Notes*. W. Wood, New York, 1870.

Echeverria MG. Marriage and hereditariness of epileptics. *J Ment Sci* 1881; 26:346–90.

Esquirol E. *Mental Maladies. A Treatise on Insanity*. Transl. Hunt EK. Lea & Blanchard, Philadelphia, 1845.

Fernelius J. *Universa Medicina*. Lutetiae Parisiorum: Paris Aput. Andream Wechelu, Frankfurt, 1567.

Gowers WR. *Epilepsy and Other Chronic Convulsive Disorders*. Churchill, London, 1881.

Gowers WR. *A Manual of Diseases of the Nervous System*. Blakiston, Philadelphia, 1888.

Gowers WR. *Epilepsy and Other Chronic Convulsive Disorders*, 2nd edn. Churchill, London, 1901.

Hippocrates. Des maladies des femmes. In *Oeuvres Completes d'Hippocrate*, Transl. Littre E, Vol. VIII: Books I, II, and VII. J. Baillière, Paris, 1839–1861.

Hippocrates *Hippocrates*. Transl. Jones WHS. Loeb Classical Library, II, 139–41. Harvard University Press, PA, 1923.

Huette G. Recherches sur les properties physiologiques et therapeutiques du bromiure de potassium. *Med Gaz Paris* 1850; 21:432.

Institoris H. *Malleus Maleficarum*. Transl. Summers M. Rodker, London, 1928.

Laforgue. Rev Medicale de Toulouse, 1867. Quoted by Echeverria, p. 321.

La Motte GM de. *Traite complet de chirurgie*, Vol. 2. Paris, 1771, p. 422.

Landouzy H. *Trait de L'Hysterie*, JB et G Baillière, Paris, 1846.

Lennox, WG with the collaboration of MA Lennox. *Epilepsy and Related Disorders*, 2 volumes. Little Brown, Boston, 1960.

Leuba JH. *The Psychology of Religious Mysticism*. Kegan Paul, Trench, Trubner, London, 1925.

Locock C. Discussion of paper by E.H. Sieveking. Analysis of fifty-two cases of epilepsy observed by the author. *Lancet* 1857; 1:527.

Maudsley H. *The Pathology of Mind.* Macmillan, London, 1879.

Maudsley H. *Physiology and Pathology of the Mind.* W. L. Kingsley, New Haven, CT, 1867.

Munson JF. The treatment of the epilepsies. In White WA, Jelliffe SE. *Modern Treatment of Nervous and Mental Diseases*, Vol. 2. Lea and Febiger, Philadelphia, 1913, pp. 225–73.

Paracelsus. *Four Treatises of Theophrastus von Hohenheim called Paracelsus.* Introductory essays by Temkin CL, Rosen G, Zilboorg G, Sigerist HE. Johns Hopkins University Press, Baltimore, 1941, pp. 163–4.

Pliny. *Naturalis historica*, rec. Janus L. Leipzig, vols. 2–6, 1856–1865; vol. 4, p. 162.

Prichard JC. *A Treatise on Diseases of the Nervous System.* Underwood, London, 1822, p. 190.

Reynolds JR. *Epilepsy: its Symptoms, Treatment, and Relation to Other Chronic Convulsive Diseases.* Churchill, London, 1861.

Schenckius a Grafenberg J. *Observationum medicarum rariorum*, libri VII. Lyon, 1644.

Scott DF. *The History of Epileptic Therapy.* Parthenon Pub, Carnforth, Iowa, 1993.

Sieveking EH. *On Epilepsy and Epileptiform Seizures: Their Causes, Pathology, and Treatment*, 2nd edn. Churchill, London, 1861.

Spratling WP. *Epilepsy and its Treatment.* WB Saunders, New York, 1904.

Temkin O. *The Falling Sickness*, 2nd edn, revised. Johns Hopkins University Press, Baltimore, 1971.

Tissot SA. *Traite de l'epilepsie.* Didot Le Jaune, Paris, 1770.

Trousseau A. *Clinique medicale de l'Hotel-Dieu de Paris*, 3rd edn, Vol. II. Paris, 1868. Cited by D'Olier.

Veith I. *Hysteria: the History of a Disease.* University of Chicago Press, Chicago, 1965.

Wilks S. Bromide and iodide of potassium in epilepsy. Cases and clinical remarks by Dr. Wilks. *Med Times Gaz* 1861; 2:635–6.

Wilson-Kinnier JV, Reynolds EH. Translation and analysis of a cuneiform text forming part of a Babylonian treatise on epilepsy. *Med Hist* 1990; 34:185–98.

4

Quality of life issues for women with epilepsy

Joyce A. Cramer

Joyce Cramer is a well-known researcher in the fields of epilepsy and psychiatry and holds an appointment at Yale University. Her recent work has focused on the quality of life for people with chronic illness, especially those with epilepsy. She was one of the developers of the Quality of Life in Epilepsy Inventory (QOLIE), which allows people with epilepsy to discuss life concerns by means of a detailed survey. She has challenged the health-care field to consider the well-being of the whole person with epilepsy rather than having a narrow focus on seizure control alone.

In this chapter, Ms Cramer discusses how quality of life may be disrupted by epilepsy and provides suggestions about how to communicate your quality of life concerns to your health-care team. Caring for the whole person works best when the person with epilepsy is an active partner in her care.

MJM

What is 'quality of life'?

Health-related quality of life (HRQOL) has been defined by the World Health Organization as a state of complete physical, mental, and social well-being, and not merely the absence of disease or infirmity. It can also be defined as the functional effect of an illness and its consequent therapy on a patient, as perceived by the patient. Within the many aspects of HRQOL, an individual person perceives a problem when there is a difference between actual and desired health status. When the gap between where we are compared to where we would like to be is wide, HRQOL is low. A woman whose epilepsy is poorly controlled, but who can maintain her home and care for her family, or enjoy a successful career, may be pleased with her life. In contrast, a child restricted from playing sports may feel like a social outcast; a teenager whose occasional seizures cause embarrassment at school and lead to a loss of friends may feel severely limited by epilepsy.

The medical profession has only recently moved toward appreciating that HRQOL is an important component in assessing the effectiveness of health care. This is particularly welcome at a time when women are becoming more aware of the options available for good medical care. The popular self-help book *Men are from Mars, Women are from Venus* describes how men and women find communicating with one another so difficult that it is as if they are from different planets. Perhaps the title should also include '*And* Doctors are from the Moon' to describe the way some health-care professionals view patient needs. This description is not a negative statement, but one that reflects the different ways that each group listens, perceives, and communicates about issues. The hallmark of HRQOL assessment is that it must reflect what the individual patient feels, and needs, not what the health-care provider thinks are the problems.

Why is epilepsy different?

Epilepsy is a condition with long periods of normal function interrupted occasionally by brief periods of seizure activity. People with epilepsy, even if they have not had a seizure for several years, carry the diagnosis without obvious signs or symptoms. Unlike people who have arthritis with daily pain, seizures *can* occur rarely. Unlike people with so-called 'silent disorders,' such as hypertension, people who are diagnosed with epilepsy have already experienced two or more seizures. They know the physical, psychological, and social impact of seizures, and cannot be guaranteed that seizure activity will not recur, even while they are in a current period of remission. These concerns underlie many of the perceived limitations related to epilepsy. Stopping seizures and discontinuing medications relieve some of the burden of being labeled as an epilepsy patient. However, some aspects of distress continue (such as fear of recurrence) long after the seizures.

Whose perceptions do we value?

Traditional assessments of social function have been made by physicians, nurses, psychologists, and social workers based on brief interviews with the patient, reports from the family, and interaction during the medical examination. This way of obtaining information places less value on what a patient actually experiences. For example, a patient who is docile when sedated by medications is considered 'demanding' by the family when physical and psychological function improves. Only the patient can tell us how he or she feels as an individual. Information from surrogates or proxies differs from what *you* can tell us about *your* daily life or level of function. The purpose of evaluating HRQOL is to determine what *you* feel, what *you* need, and what *you* want.

What issues comprise the scope of quality of life?

Five general domains can be used to describe HRQOL:
1 physical condition
2 psychological condition
3 vocational (work) capacity
4 social function
5 disease-specific conditions.

Physical issues

Not only can severe seizures cause injury from falling, but mild seizures can also lead to danger during periods of altered consciousness. In addition, treatment with antiepileptic drugs often brings unwanted 'side effects,' particularly when it is necessary to raise the dose of medication to maximal tolerance in order to control seizures. The balance between adverse effects and seizure control may have different meanings for the patient and the physician. How much distress and discomfort should be tolerated from drug-related adverse effects? Adverse effects may be dose related or idiosyncratic (individual response). You may be able to help with the adjustment of dose-related effects by determining which are bothersome and which require immediate dose reduction to alleviate the problem. Idiosyncratic effects are more difficult to anticipate and modify, but may also need your assessment of tolerability.

Psychological issues

People commonly experience depression at the time of the initial diagnosis of epilepsy and this mood change can be prolonged or chronic. The feeling of not being in control of one's health and resentment of the need to take medication may be major factors, often leading to noncompliance with a medication regimen. Testing the diagnosis by discontinuing or reducing medication intake is common, particularly in disorders such as epilepsy, in which seizure recurrence is not necessarily immediate. The positive feedback gained by the person who omits doses without having immediate seizures may have an important negative influence on the later ability to readjust to a medication schedule if seizures recur. The effects of medication and seizures also may impinge on psychological well-being, particularly if cognition is impaired or memory loss becomes apparent to the patient. Evaluation with neuropsychological tests can help the neurologist decide how severe problems are and whether they are new or long-standing.

Vocational issues

Whether or not a person with epilepsy is working depends not only on her capacity for a specific type of work but also on her availability for that work. For example, a woman may have directed an independent accounting firm, but may become unable to perform at that level because of slowed thinking or frequent seizures. Taking a job as an accountant near home, at half the usual wage, would count as full-time employment. Nonetheless, the level of employment is far lower than her qualifications and aspirations. The fact that a person is able and willing to work full time, but is actually working only part time, or at a lower-level position, indicates a reduced level of vocational function in terms of both salary and status. Employability is not necessarily related to seizure frequency. Some people are able to work despite frequent seizures, whereas others cannot become employed after successful surgery to stop seizures. Enactment of the Americans With Disabilities Act of 1990 should help people with epilepsy obtain employment and maintain jobs, with special accommodation provided by employers.

Social issues

Social function is often impaired because of the stigma associated with a diagnosis of epilepsy (Table 4.1). Relationships within the family may change, with less responsibility given to the woman with epilepsy. Relationships with friends and coworkers are also affected, particularly when they have witnessed you having a seizure. Just when you most need friendship, you may find that friends are no longer willing to give you a ride in their car or invite

Table 4.1. Aspects of epilepsy that often lead to social withdrawal

Seizures
    Type (e.g., maintain awareness, warning)
    Frequency
Medication effects
    Overt (e.g., tremor, sedation)
    Subtle (e.g., cognition, memory)
Employment
    Unemployment
    Underemployment
    Restricted employment
Psychological
    Anxiety (e.g., fear of exposure of diagnosis)
    Lack of control (e.g., recurrence of seizures)
    Dependency
    Depression
    Self-esteem
Social
    Limited social contacts
    Limited financial resources
    Low marriage/fertility rates
Stigma of epilepsy
    Perceived (e.g., hide diagnosis)
    Actual (e.g., restricted opportunities)

you into their home for fear that you will have a seizure in their presence. The seemingly minor limitations in your lifestyle, ranging from restrictions for a child's play, an adolescent's driving, an adult's drinking alcohol, may mark you as 'different' because you have epilepsy. Whether restrictions and stigma are real or perceived, if you feel the social constraints, then you are limited by the diagnosis of epilepsy. The good news is that lifestyle can improve significantly when seizures become controlled. Removal of driving restrictions and of restrictions on sports and work activities and reduced burden of medications (both dosing and side effects) can allow a semi-reclusive adult or closely supervised child to become 'normalized.' However, just as the cancer survivor worries about recurrence for years, it is not unusual for the

Table 4.2. Uses of a QOLIE assessment

Does what?
Assesses issues
Develops concepts
Implements therapy
Evaluates changes
For whom?
Patient
Physician
Physician and patient
How?
Defines personal problems and needs
Gives specifics on patient needs
Focuses attention on remediable issues
Clarifies follow-up

fear that seizures will restart to continue for years after becoming seizure free.

Disease-specific issues

The hallmark of epilepsy is the occurrence of seizures, but there are many types of seizures that vary in severity. How many seizures are too many? For some, even one seizure is too many. The person who improves from having weekly seizures to just one seizure every few months will feel markedly improved. However, over time, this person also may begin to consider the possibility of even better seizure control. It is up to the individual to question the possibility of further improvement so the health-care providers continue to consider new therapies.

How can we evaluate HRQOL in epilepsy?

Several questionnaires have been developed that allow people with epilepsy to express their concerns about the variety of issues that affect their lives (Table 4.2). The QOLIE instruments were developed as measures of quality of life in epilepsy with three separate questionnaires. The most extensive measure, the QOLIE-89, contains 89 items grouped into 17 multi-item scales (and three single items). The 17 scales can be grouped into four dimensions: (1) epilepsy-targeted, (2) cognitive, (3) mental health, and (4) physical health. Two shorter instruments have also been developed, containing subsets of items in the QOLIE-89. The QOLIE-31 has 31 items grouped into seven multi-item scales. A ten-item screening tool (QOLIE-10) was derived from the QOLIE-31. QOLIE scores show distinct differences among groups of people with varying severity of epilepsy. Those with more frequent and severe seizures have worse QOLIE scores than people who are well controlled.

Each questionnaire is designed for easy response. The major differences among the questionnaires are the number of issues covered in various sub-scales, with several questions related to each issue. The QOLIE-89 is the most comprehensive questionnaire (covering 17 areas), and the QOLIE-31 covers just seven areas thought to be most important to people with epilepsy. The QOLIE-10 covers the same seven subscales, but with just one question for each issue (Table 4.3).

All of the questionnaires can be scored to provide sub-scale scores and an overall, total QOLIE score. The importance of having a standardized questionnaire is that these numbers can be used for comparison among groups, or to look at differences in how an individual responds from time to time. Neurologists and specialized epilepsy centers are beginning to use the QOLIE questionnaires as part of routine patient assessment. Even the QOLIE-10, completed in just a few minutes in the waiting room, can provide important information for the health-care team because it defines what areas are problems for someone on a particular day. Even if your doctor does not review the QOLIE, it might be useful for you to complete a questionnaire to familiarize yourself with the types of issues that are common for people with epilepsy. Sometimes, just knowing that you are not the only person who is concerned about certain issues is helpful. For example, children commonly fear that they will die during a seizure, but are unable to express that fear without direct questioning. Getting the fear out in the open in a discussion with the health-care team usually relieves the tension surrounding such fears and worries. In that way, the QOLIE might help you bring specific questions into your next discussion with the health-care team.

Table 4.3. The 17 subscales demonstrating the areas covered by the QOLIE

Health perceptions
Seizure worry*
Physical function
Role limitation – physical
Role limitation – emotional
Pain
Overall quality of life*
Emotional well-being*
Energy/fatigue*
Attention/concentration*
Memory
Language
Medication effects*
Social function, work, driving*
Social support
Social isolation
Health discouragement
Sexual function
Change in health
Overall health*

Items marked with an asterisk are included in the abbreviated QOLIE-31 and QOLIE-10

What can the neurologist do to improve quality of life for patients?

The use of HRQOL assessment as part of routine assessment for people with epilepsy gives them the opportunity to respond to direct questions about all major aspects of living with epilepsy. This approach assists the health-care providers to expand beyond the traditional issues of the number of seizures experienced and the type of side effects caused by medications to the other lifestyle issues you deal with day to day. You can change the major focus of encounters with doctors from tests and numbers to you and your level of function. As health-care professionals learn how to ask about and use HRQOL information, they learn which special resources in a community are needed to assist an individual. Social agencies might also provide information directly to you, further enhancing your role in self-care.

How are HRQOL assessments used?

There are several medical uses for HRQOL information. They can be used to alert the health-care team to someone's specific concerns, inform patients of problems common for this disorder, and assist both patients and their doctors in making decisions. HRQOL questionnaires can provide a baseline score for comparison of change over time. Level of function can improve or worsen after a change in drug dose or medication, use of another intervention such as surgery, or the emergence of other medical problems. Equally important issues related to social function, employment, and psychological state (e.g., depression, mental speed) could also affect quality of life without noticeably affecting medical assessments. HRQOL scores can be considered a new measure of overall patient function, like blood levels for antiepileptic drugs.

Conclusion

HRQOL is a new name for a common-sense approach to working with the needs of every individual, as identified by the individuals themselves. Epilepsy is a disorder that you can live with. Make the most of your life.

SELECTED REFERENCES

Cramer JA. Quality of life for people with epilepsy. Neurologic Clinics: Epilepsy II: Special Issues, ed. O Devinsky. WB Saunders Company, New York, 1994; 12:1–13.

Cramer JA. Compliance and quality of life. In *Epilepsy and Quality of Life*, ed. MR Trimble, WE Dodson. Raven Press, New York, 1994, pp. 49–63.

Cramer JA. Quality of life assessments in epilepsy. In *Quality of Life and Pharmacoeconomics in Clinical Trials*, ed. B Spilker. Lippincott-Raven Publishers, Philadelphia, 1996, pp. 909–18.

Cramer JA, Perrine K, Devinsky O, Bryant-Comstock L, Meador K, Hermann B. Development and cross-cultural translations of a 31-Item Quality of Life in epilepsy inventory. *Epilepsia* 1998; **39**(1):81–8.

Cramer JA, Perrine K, Devinsky O, Meador K. A brief questionnaire to screen for quality of life in epilepsy: The QOLIE-10. *Epilepsia* 1996; 37:577–82.

Devinsky O, Vickrey BG, Perrine K, et al. Development of an instrument of health-related quality of life for people with epilepsy. *Epilepsia* 1995; 36:1089–104.

Jacoby A. Epilepsy and the quality of everyday life: findings from a study of people with well-controlled epilepsy. *Soc Sci Med* 1992; 34:657–66.

Vickrey BG, Hays RD, Graber J, Rausch R, Engel J, Brook RH. A health-related quality of life instrument for patients evaluated for epilepsy surgery. *Med Care* 1992; 30:299–319.

Part II

Epilepsy diagnosis and treatment

5

The genetics of epilepsy

Melodie R. Winawer and Ruth Ottman

Medical research will soon identify the genetic causes of some epilepsies. As epilepsy genes are identified, therapies will be developed that directly target the specific cause of the epilepsy. Such treatments will provide better seizure control and even epilepsy cures. Tests will also be developed so that parents can be counseled regarding the risk of transmitting epilepsy to their offspring.

What we know so far indicates that many epilepsies are genetic and that there are many genes that can cause epilepsy. To find epilepsy genes, researchers must identify families with genetic epilepsies, and then perform a gene analysis in each individual in order to find the common epilepsy gene. This type of research depends on the generosity of individuals with epilepsy and their family members, who participate by allowing medical researchers to gather seizure information and to collect blood samples. In order to make it easier for people with epilepsy to participate in epilepsy gene research, while maintaining strict confidentiality of medical information, the Epilepsy Foundation has developed the Gene Discovery Project. This allows family trees (pedigrees) to be entered into an anonymous website. This information can then be made available to researchers in epilepsy. The Epilepsy Foundation contacts individuals whose family information is of interest to a particular researcher and provides details about how the investigator can be contacted. More information about the Gene Discovery Project is available on the Epilepsy Foundation website (*www.epilepsyfoundation.org*).

Dr Ottman is a Professor in the School of Public Health at Columbia University. She is an established medical scientist who has conducted research into the genetic basis of epilepsy. Her colleague, Dr Winawer, is an Assistant Professor of Neurology and has recently received funding from the National Institutes of Health to look for the genes underlying some specific types of seizures. This chapter provides an overview of epilepsy and genetics that is thorough and comprehensible.

MJM

Recent advances in research are helping scientists, doctors, and patients to have a better understanding of the way genes affect the risk for epilepsy.

Several specific genes have been discovered that raise the risk for developing certain types of epilepsy – but most epilepsy is still not explained by known genes. The identification of epilepsy genes can contribute in many more important ways to public and individual health. It can allow the early identification of people at risk for developing epilepsy, and may eventually lead to the development of methods to prevent the onset of epilepsy in these individuals. Also, discovery of these genes can contribute to a better understanding of the process by which the brain becomes susceptible to seizures, leading to the development of new strategies for treatment and prevention in the future.

General information about epilepsy

In order to understand the genetic causes of epilepsy, it is important to review a few basic concepts and definitions. Epilepsy is a disorder in which seizures occur repeatedly, without any immediate cause. In about 25% of cases, a past injury to the brain (more than a week before the first seizure) is likely to have caused the epilepsy, even though there is no *immediate* cause of the seizures. Epilepsy with an identifiable injury to the brain (e.g., head trauma, stroke, or brain infection) is called symptomatic epilepsy. In the remaining 75% of those affected, the cause is unknown – epilepsy with unknown cause is called either idiopathic (which means of 'unknown' cause) or cryptogenic (which means of 'hidden' cause).

Epilepsy is highly variable, with many different types of seizures, ages at onset, responses to treatment, and other features. For this reason, we sometimes refer to 'the epilepsies,' to indicate that this is a group of disorders, many of which may have different causes, rather than a single disease or condition. The epilepsies are classified according to seizure type and epilepsy syndrome into the following categories.

- Generalized seizures are seizures that involve the entire brain (both sides) from the outset. Some examples of generalized seizures are absence, myoclonic, atonic, and generalized tonic–clonic (also called primary generalized grand mal).
- Absence seizures are sometimes called petit mal because they appear to be simply staring spells with no convulsive movements.

- Partial (or focal) seizures begin in a specific area of the brain. Partial seizures many then spread to involve the whole brain, in which a secondarily generalized grand mal seizure occurs, but partial seizures may also stay in just one part of the brain.
- An epileptic syndrome is an epileptic disorder characterized by a cluster of signs and symptoms, which usually occur together. A syndrome can include features such as type of seizure, cause, precipitating factors, severity, age of onset, and prognosis.
- Generalized epilepsy syndromes are epilepsy syndromes characterized by generalized seizures.
- Localization-related epilepsy syndromes are syndromes characterized by partial or focal seizures.

Basic genetics: terms and concepts

Genes

Genes are the basic units of inheritance. They are made of a chemical called deoxyribonucleic acid (DNA). Human beings have about 100 000 genes, and each of these genes influences one or more specific traits. For example, there are genes that affect eye color, hair color, blood type, and many other characteristics. People differ with respect to these traits because their genes are different. However, many traits are partially influenced by genes and partially by the environment and sometimes it is difficult to tell whether a given characteristic is determined by genes, the environment, or a combination of both. For example, people may be born with a certain hair color, but change their natural hair color by using dyes, thus making their genetic hair color unclear.

Chromosomes

Chromosomes are cellular bodies composed of DNA and other substances. Humans have 23 pairs of chromosomes (total chromosomes 46). One member of each pair comes from the mother and the other from the father. This is the basis for the inheritance of genetically determined traits from parents to their children. The genes are located on the chromosomes, arranged in a precise linear order – like houses on a street (Fig. 5.1). Each specific gene is located on the same chromosome, in the same position, in all individuals. If

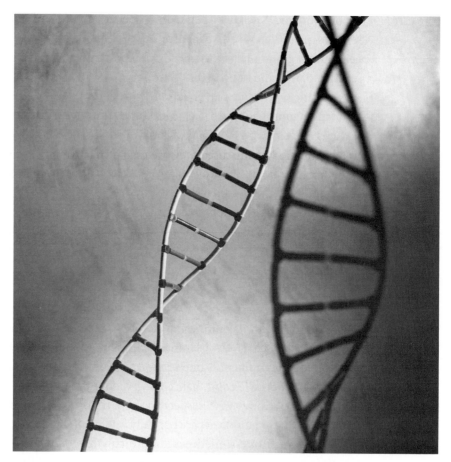

Figure 5.1   Deoxyribonucleic acid (DNA) helix – the building block of genes.

genes are altered, they may sometimes result in disease. These altered genes, called mutations, can be passed on to offspring and cause disease in later generations.

Some characteristics are inherited from single genes; these are called 'simple' genetic traits. Most epilepsy is probably not caused by single genes, although a few rare types of epilepsy have been found to result from a single altered gene. There are several patterns, or modes, of single gene inheritance: autosomal dominant, autosomal recessive, X-linked dominant, and X-linked recessive.

Autosomal dominant disease

In an autosomal dominant disease, an individual is affected if he or she carries either one or two copies of the disease gene. This means that only one copy of the abnormal gene – inherited either from the mother or the father – is sufficient to produce disease (100% of the time) in the child. In autosomal dominant diseases, the trait appears in every generation, and the risk of developing the disease is 50% in parents, siblings, and children of a person who has the disease. More distant relatives are at lower risk of developing the disease. Unaffected individuals (those who do not have the disease) cannot transmit the trait to their children in autosomal dominant inheritance. Several rare forms of epilepsy have been discovered in a few families that have autosomal dominant inheritance. Benign familial neonatal convulsions, a genetic syndrome affecting newborns, is one such disease. Most epilepsy is not autosomal dominant, however.

Autosomal recessive disease

Autosomal recessive genes cause disease only if a person receives two copies of the disease gene (one from each parent). The disease usually occurs only in siblings of the affected person, and approximately one-quarter of siblings are affected. Several rare diseases that cause severe mental retardation, epilepsy, and other neurological problems are inherited in an autosomal recessive manor. Progressive myoclonic epilepsy (Unverricht–Lundborg disease) is one example of an autosomal recessive seizure disorder.

Sex chromosomes

Two of the 46 total human chromosomes are called sex chromosomes. Sex chromosomes come in two types, X and Y. In humans, gender is determined by the presence or absence of the Y chromosome. Individuals with two X chromosomes are female, and those with one X and one Y chromosome are male. If a gene is located on the X chromosome, it is called X-linked.

X-linked dominant disease

In an X-linked dominant disease, only one copy of the disease gene is necessary to cause disease in both males and females. X-linked lissencephaly (classical lissencephaly) is one example of an X-linked dominant disease, with severe mental retardation and epilepsy.

X-linked recessive disease

In an X-linked recessive disease, males are affected if they carry a single copy of the disease gene on their single X chromosome, whereas females are affected only if they carry two copies of the disease gene, one on each of their two X chromosomes. Because it is more likely that someone will inherit one than two copies of a gene, X-linked diseases are much more common in males than in females. Affected males inherit the disease from their mothers, who are 'asymptomatic carriers.' In other words, women without symptoms of the disorder carry a disease gene that they can pass on to their children.

Most epilepsy does not follow these simple patterns of inheritance. However, studying the rare types with these patterns can help us understand more about the causes of epilepsy and its genetic complexity.

Questions and answers

Is epilepsy inherited?

The answer to this question is quite complicated, for several reasons. First, epilepsy is not a single disorder, but instead a collection of many different disorders linked by the common fact that they result in recurrent, unprovoked seizures. Therefore, some epilepsies are more likely to be influenced by genetics than others and, even among genetically determined epilepsies, the genes responsible will vary. In addition, most epilepsy is *not* determined by simple modes of inheritance in which there is a clear, predictable relationship between having an altered gene and developing a disorder. When inheritance of a specific gene is not sufficient to cause disease, some gene carriers will be unaffected. This is called reduced penetrance. In this case, other genes or environmental factors may be needed for the specific gene to cause disease. Genetic and nongenetic factors (such as head injury) may work together to produce seizures. This phenomenon is known as gene–environment interaction. Alternatively, multiple genes may work together to increase the risk of developing epilepsy.

Even when two individuals may appear to have the same type of epilepsy or epilepsy syndrome, they may have it as a result of different causes. For example, two brothers may both have epilepsy with generalized tonic–clonic (grand mal) seizures, one as a result of a genetic cause, and the other as a result of head trauma. This is called etiologic heterogeneity, meaning resulting from different causes. Because the relationship between genes and the development of seizures is so complex, instead of saying 'epilepsy is inherited,' it is more accurate to say that 'risk of epilepsy is influenced by genes.'

What is the risk that epilepsy will develop in family members of people with epilepsy?

Overall, there is good evidence indicating that epilepsy does run in families. However, it is important to realize that the great majority of people with epilepsy – approximately 90% – do not have any affected relatives. Different studies have shown that the risk of epilepsy in brothers, sisters, and children of individuals with epilepsy ranges from 4–8%, compared with a risk in the general population of 1–2%. Although risks are clearly elevated in family members of individuals with epilepsy when compared to the general population, the numbers are actually low: most people with epilepsy have no affected relatives, and the majority of parents with epilepsy do not have children with epilepsy.

The risk of developing epilepsy in the relatives of affected people is increased compared with the general population, but the size of this risk depends on many factors. One factor is the closeness of the relationship to the affected person. Parents, brothers, sisters, and children of individuals with epilepsy are at greater risk than more distant relatives such as aunts, uncles, or cousins. The clinical features of the epilepsy, including age at onset of seizures and epilepsy type have also been shown to affect risk to relatives (see the next question).

Which types of epilepsy are most likely to be inherited?
Generalized versus localization-related epilepsy

The risk to family members depends on the kind of epilepsy an individual has. In the close relatives (parents, brothers, sisters, and children) of patients with generalized epilepsy, the risk of epilepsy is higher than in the close relatives of people with localization-related (partial or focal) epilepsy. One particular type of generalized epilepsy, absence epilepsy (often called petit mal), seems to have a particularly strong genetic influence. Several studies have shown that the risk of relatives of patients with absence seizures is higher than for other generalized or partial seizure types.

Symptomatic epilepsy versus idiopathic or cryptogenic epilepsy

Genetic risk does not appear to play a significant role in causing epilepsy in people with serious brain injuries that occurred after birth, such as head injuries, brain tumors, strokes, or brain infection (i.e., symptomatic epilepsy). This means that the risk of developing epilepsy is not increased in the relatives of someone with epilepsy resulting from these types of injuries.

Early-onset versus late-onset epilepsy

The effect of genetic factors on the risk of epilepsy decreases as people get older. After the age of 35, there is no definite effect of genetic factors on the risk. Certain specific epilepsy syndromes begin at specific ages. For example, benign rolandic epilepsy (childhood epilepsy that often remits at puberty) usually begins in children between the ages of 5 and 10 years, whereas benign familial neonatal convulsions begin shortly after birth. The onset of genetic epilepsies is not limited to children, but is unlikely to occur after young adulthood.

In keeping with this finding, the relatives of individuals whose epilepsy began early in life have a greater risk of developing epilepsy than the relatives of those with later onset epilepsy.

Febrile seizures

A febrile seizure is a type of seizure that occurs in infants or young children, usually between 3 months and 5 years of age, and is associated with fever, without evidence of nervous system infection or other direct cause of the seizure other than the fever itself. Febrile seizures are also, like epilepsy, probably a combination of disorders, not just one simple disease, and this makes the search for genetic or other causes difficult. This risk of febrile seizures is increased in the siblings and offspring of individuals with febrile seizures. The risk of epilepsy is also increased in the relatives of people with febrile convulsions, and *vice versa*.

Do mothers and fathers with epilepsy have different risks of having children with epilepsy?

Studies have shown that the risk of epilepsy is approximately twice as high in the children of women with epilepsy than in the children of men with epilepsy. So far, studies indicate that this 'maternal effect' is not due to pregnancy or birth complications, and not due to antiepileptic medications or maternal seizures. More research is underway to investigate this finding.

What type of research is being done today on genes and epilepsy?

Studying the families of people affected with epilepsy is an important way of investigating the genetic contributions to the development of epilepsy. Familial aggregation studies, which examine the way in which seizure disorders cluster in families, and twin studies, which examine the risk of epilepsy in one twin when the other is affected, provide evidence for the genetic influences on epilepsy. Studies of gene localization and identification are another important research method. The discovery of genes that raise the risk of epilepsy not only proves that the disease is genetic, but also helps us to understand how, biologically, the brain becomes susceptible to seizures.

The method most commonly used to find the chromosomal location of epilepsy genes is called linkage analysis. When we say we want to 'find' a gene that causes epilepsy, we mean that we want to determine its precise chromosomal location (its 'street address'). This is a first step in identifying the gene itself, and in discovering how a change in the gene causes epilepsy. Basically, this method involves using blood samples to look for differences in the DNA between people with and without epilepsy within families.

Which of the 100 000 human genes has been shown to influence the risk of epilepsy, and where are these genes located?

The genes that have been discovered to date are responsible for relatively rare forms of epilepsy. These syndromes include benign familial neonatal convulsions, progressive myoclonus epilepsy of Unverricht–Lundborg type, Lafora's disease, autosomal dominant nocturnal frontal lobe epilepsy, and generalized epilepsy with febrile seizures.

Future directions and implications

Although there is clear evidence that genes play an important role in raising the risk for epilepsy, for the majority of patients the specific genetic influences have still not yet been identified. The discovery of genes that cause epilepsy can help us understand more about the biological processes in the brain that affect the risk of seizures. These discoveries may also enable us to recognize patients at risk for seizures, and to start treatment early. In addition, this understanding may one day lead to the development of completely new treatments and possibly even strategies to prevent epilepsy before it begins.

SELECTED REFERENCES

Anderson VE, Andermann E, Hauser WA. Genetic counseling. In *Epilepsy: a Comprehensive Textbook*, ed. J Engel Jr, TA Pedley. Lippincott-Raven Publishers, Philadelphia, 1997, 225–32.

Anderson VE, Hauser WA, Rich SS. Genetic Heterogeneity in the Epilepsies. Advances in Neurology; Vol 44. Delgado-Escueta AV, Ward AA Jr., Woodbury DM, and Porter RJ, Eds. Raven Press, New York, 1986.

Annegers JF, Hauser WA, Anderson VE, Kurland LT. The risks of seizure disorders among relatives of patients with childhood onset epilepsy. *Neurology* 1982; 32:174–9.

Ottman R. Genetic epidemiology of epilepsy. *Epidemiol Rev* 1997; 19:120–8.

Thompson MW, McInnes RR, Willard HF. Thompson & Thompson: *Genetics in Medicine*, 5th edn. WB Saunders, Philadelphia, 1991.

6

Epilepsy: epidemiology, definitions, and diagnostic procedures

Simon Shorvon and Dominic Heaney

Dr Dominic Heaney and Professor Simon Shorvon are epilepsy specialists at the National Hospital for Neurology and Neurosurgery and the National Society for Epilepsy in London, England. They provide an overview of epilepsy, discussing its causes, the frequency with which it occurs throughout the world, definitions of the various types of seizures, and a review of the tests that are used for diagnosis and to monitor response to treatment.

Professor Shorvon is an internationally known expert in the field of epilepsy and serves as editor of the official publication of the International League Against Epilepsy. He is therefore able to provide a valuable international perspective.

As Dr Heaney and Professor Shorvon discuss, epilepsy may go undiagnosed and untreated, especially in the developing world, where access to medical care is limited. The burden of epilepsy is also great in the developed world. In the USA, the cost of epilepsy is 12.2 billion dollars a year. Only 15% of this is related to direct medical costs (doctors, tests, medications). Eighty-five percent is in 'indirect costs' such as missed educational opportunities, underemployment, and unemployment. Unemployment affects 25% of people with epilepsy in the USA, and this is likely to be a particular problem for women.

MJM

Introduction

Epilepsy is one of the most common neurological conditions throughout the world. Despite this, it remains a 'hidden' condition and people who develop it can feel isolated and stigmatized. For many patients, it is important to discover how many other people are affected and then to understand the many different definitions, classifications, and causes of epilepsy that are likely to be described. This chapter describes these areas by outlining and defining the epidemiology and etiology of epilepsy and explains how these issues are closely related to the present systems of defining and classifying epilepsy. Issues particularly relevant to women are highlighted. Finally, the major techniques used to investigate epilepsy are described.

Epidemiology

Epilepsy is hidden, rarely talked about, and is often regarded with fear and prejudice by individuals, organizations, and governments throughout the world. Outside of the medical community, there is little understanding about the different *types* of epilepsy and, for most, epilepsy is synonymous with generalized tonic–clonic convulsion. A poignant example of the public's lack of sympathy can be seen when one considers the voluntary contributions made to charities. In the UK in 1996, voluntary contributions to the two main epilepsy charities amounted to £2.1 million – for a condition that affects nearly half a million people at any one time, and may affect up to 5% of the British population at some time in their lives. In comparison, motor neuron disease, a condition that affects only a few thousand people per year, attracted charitable donations of £2.2 million. Multiple sclerosis charities received £11.9 million and a single UK animal charity received £18.7 million.

Epidemiological studies are those that describe the pattern of disease within populations. Large studies have been performed in many countries around the world and have greatly enhanced the understanding of epilepsy. Epidemiological studies not only provide information about the incidence (the number of new cases) and prevalence (number of people with the condition) of epilepsy, but also help identify factors that may be important causes of it. Nevertheless, the public's lack of understanding and occasional hostility toward epilepsy make the task of epidemiologists very difficult. In order to perform such studies, it is essential to identify correctly all cases of epilepsy. This is not easy when individuals with epilepsy may hide themselves or may even fail to realize that they are suffering from epilepsy. Additional problems arise because of the varied ways in which epilepsy may manifest itself. Seizures can vary from prolonged, severe, generalized tonic–clonic convulsions, to very brief 'partial' seizures, in which consciousness is barely affected. The identification of people with epilepsy is straightforward when they are suffering frequent generalized seizures, but far more difficult when seizures are more subtle and may not be recognized by the individual or her family. For example, many patients with myoclonic jerks and absence seizures do not recognize their symptoms as being caused by epilepsy. It should be realized that most studies show that less than 40% of patients have generalized seizures. In other words, 60% of people with epilepsy have seizures that may not be easily recognized.

Not withstanding these difficulties, several excellent epidemiological studies have been performed in a large number of developing and developed countries. Key features of epilepsy have been identified, which have given insight into the likely causes and prognosis of the condition. One of the main observations is the extraordinary heterogeneity of epilepsy.

On average, in a population of 1 million people, there will be up to 10 000 people with epilepsy and 1000 new cases will appear each year. The total lifetime 'risk' of developing epilepsy can be as high as 5%. Behind these startlingly high 'headline' figures for the incidence and prevalence of epilepsy are marked variations between developed and developing countries and, in addition, demographic and secular trends have also been observed.

Most new cases of epilepsy occur in the young (less than 20 years old) and the old (greater than 65 years old). As many as two-thirds of patients will go into remission on treatment, and epilepsy can be described as inactive if a patient has not suffered a seizure for 5 years or more. There is no great gender difference in the frequency of epilepsy – women are just as likely to develop epilepsy as men.

There are geographical variations in the incidence and prevalence of epilepsy. Studies have shown that populations in developing countries are more likely to have a greater incidence of epilepsy than those in the richer West. Moreover, prevalence rates are higher than those seen in developed countries such as the USA or Europe.

Epidemiological studies have also demonstrated that people with epilepsy suffer a higher mortality rate than those without epilepsy. Overall, this risk is thought to be two to three times higher than that of the 'normal' population. Most of this excess risk occurs within the first 10 years following diagnosis, and males are more likely to die than females. In part, this increased mortality rate is due to the underlying causes of some of the epilepsies (such as brain tumors or cerebrovascular disease), but its full explanation is still being researched.

Overall, the epidemiological profiles of epilepsy in men and women are similar. There are, of course, exceptions. Certain rarer epileptic syndromes are more common in one sex than the other and there are differences in the 'epidemiology' of risk factors for epilepsy (such as road traffic accidents and head injury).

Pathology

One of the most common questions asked by people who have epilepsy is 'what caused it?'. The 'causes of epilepsy' can be considered on two levels. First, how is the normal central nervous system physiology disrupted to the extent that epileptic seizures occur? Second, what is the underlying problem that causes some individuals to be affected but not others? It should be understood that although the major 'symptom' in epilepsy – an epileptic seizure – can appear to be very similar in different individuals, there are a huge number of different causes for epilepsy.

In a person without epilepsy, neurons (nerve cells) within the central nervous system discharge repetitively at a low baseline frequency and it is this controlled electrical activity that can be measured using an electroencephalograph (EEG). Epileptic seizures are produced by an abnormal rhythmic and repetitive discharge of neurons, either localized to a particular part of the brain (the 'focal' area) or 'generalized' throughout the whole cerebral cortex. In many cases, these abnormal discharges can be detected with an EEG. The precise reason why some seizures are limited to certain areas of the brain whereas others 'generalize', affecting the whole brain, is not well understood. It is likely that local brain cell chemicals play a part in inhibiting the spread of seizures.

In most people with epilepsy, seizures occur in a completely random fashion and are totally unpredictable. However, some patients are able to identify certain common precipitants that may trigger their seizures. Examples of these may include fatigue, stress, emotionally charged situations, or flickering lights. Approximately 60% of women notice that their seizures are worse at the time of their menstrual period. When women suffer seizures only at the time of their period, their epilepsy is described as 'catamenial'. The relationship between the menstrual cycle and seizures is not fully understood and may relate to an increase in levels of estrogen relative to progesterone, a decrease in the level of antiepileptic drugs in the bloodstream, fluid and electrolyte imbalance, or even increased psychological stress associated with premenstrual tension. Unfortunately, hormonal treatments have little effect, although progesterone has been reported to be associated with a decrease in seizures in some women.

Pathologies and etiologies

The likely cause of a patient's epilepsy depends on her age and the type of seizures from which she suffers. A child may suffer brain damage during the mother's pregnancy or at birth as a result of infection, trauma, metabolic disturbances, or hypoxia (a lack of oxygen to cells). Malformations of cortical development during pregnancy may also be associated with a tendency toward seizures. 'Febrile seizures' are a specific type of seizure that occur in children aged between 6 months and 5 years during the early stages of a febrile illness (the state of having a fever). The prognosis is excellent when these seizures are short, nonrecurrent, are not associated with a background of neurological handicap, and have not been caused by an infection of the central nervous system. Adolescents develop the syndrome of epilepsy described as idiopathic (of unknown cause) or primary generalized epilepsy. In this syndrome, patients often have a family history of generalized epilepsy, suggesting that genetic factors are important, and the seizure types seen are generalized tonic–clonic seizures, typical absence seizures, and myoclonic seizures, on their own or in different combinations. Patients often have a typical EEG pattern, but it is rarely possible to identify any specific pathological findings or 'cause' for this epilepsy, and this can be very distressing for patients and their families seeking to understand the condition.

Important causes of adult epilepsy include cerebrovascular disease, head injury, alcohol abuse, and central nervous system 'brain' tumors. In developing countries, cerebral infections such neurocystercicosis and malaria are frequent causes of epilepsy. Adults may also develop idiopathic epilepsy or epilepsy that is caused by pathologies developed in childhood.

Genetics

Many people suspect a genetic cause for their epilepsy and are afraid that they might pass it on to their children. However, the 'inheritance' of the condition depends very much on the type of epilepsy an individual suffers. Some types of epilepsy have a clear genetic basis and these tend to be associated with more widespread neurological disease. They include tuberous sclerosis, fragile X, and the mitochondrial encephalopathies. Gene mapping has established a strong genetic basis for three specific epilepsy syndromes: benign neonatal convulsions, juvenile myoclonic epilepsy, and the Unverricht–Lundborg form of progressive myoclonic epilepsy. The genetic link is weaker in idiopathic epilepsy, and in other epilepsies the link is even less clear. Interestingly, the risk of 'passing on' epilepsy between generations is higher when the mother is affected (8.7% versus 2.4% when the father alone is affected). The 'baseline' risk for a child with epilepsy having a family history of epilepsy is approximately 1%.

Classification

Despite recent advances, specialists are still far from devising a system of classification for epilepsy that is based on pathological or etiological findings. This contrasts with many other medical conditions, such as anemia or breathlessness, for which a patient's illness can be classified in terms of its cause, such as 'iron deficiency anemia' or 'breathlessness resulting from left ventricular dysfunction.' Instead, classifications of epilepsy are based on the nature of the seizure.

One of the most useful systems of classification was developed in 1981 by a commission of the International League Against Epilepsy (Table 6.1). This classification divides epilepsy according to whether the seizure's onset is focal (partial) or generalized. The nature of the onset of a seizure may be clear from the description that a patient gives of the seizure or may require careful EEG investigation.

In partial seizures, patients do not usually lose consciousness. Further distinctions are made by dividing partial seizures into simple partial, complex partial, and partial attacks that 'secondarily generalize.' Simple partial seizures are epileptic events in which consciousness is fully preserved and in which the discharge usually remains localized. The clinical manifestations of a simple partial attack depend on the cortical area in which the discharge occurs. These may include involuntary motor disturbances, autonomic changes, sensory experiences, or even psychic feelings, which a patient may find very difficult to describe. Simple partial seizures usually assume the same form in an individual patient. In complex partial seizures, consciousness may be impaired and a witness may describe the patient as having

Table 6.1. International League Against Epilepsy guidelines for seizure-type classification

I	**Partial seizures** (seizures beginning locally)

A Simple partial seizures (consciousness not impaired)
1 With motor symptoms
2 With somatosensory or special sensory problems
3 With autonomic symptoms
4 With psychic symptoms

B Complex partial seizures (with impairment of consciousness)
1 Beginning as simple partial seizures and progressing to impairment of consciousness
  a With no other features
  b With features as in A.1–4
  c With automatisms

2 With impairment of consciouness at onset
  a With no other features
  b With features as in A.1–4
  c With automatisms

C Partial seizures secondarily generalized

II **Generalized seizures** (bilaterally symmetrical and without focal onset)

A 1 Absence seizures
  2 Atypical absence seizures

B Myoclonic seizures

C Clonic seizures

D Tonic seizures

E Tonic–clonic seizures

F Atonic seizures

III **Unclassified epileptic seizures** (inadequate or incomplete data)

Epilepsia 1981; 22:489–501.

become 'unresponsive' rather than unconscious. Complex partial seizures may start as a simple partial seizure, often described as the 'aura.' During a complex partial seizure, patients may perform strange and apparently confused behaviors. These may include lip-smacking or chewing movements, grimacing, undressing, and the carrying out of purposeless activities – including wandering around. Complex partial seizures usually resolve quickly, but are followed by a period of confusion. Alternatively, they may progress to a secondarily generalized seizure.

Generalized seizures are characterized by the simultaneous involvement of the whole cortex at their onset. These attacks probably begin in deep areas of the brain and project to both brain hemispheres simultaneously. There are many different types of generalized seizures. Tonic–clonic seizures, or convulsive seizures, are common. They are often referred to as 'grand mal' attacks. There is no warning (unless the seizure is a partial attack with secondary generalization) and a patient will become stiff, often crying out. The patient will lose consciousness and have no memory of the event. Clonic movements occur involving most muscles, followed by brief periods of muscle relaxation. During a tonic–clonic seizure, patients may bite their tongue, salivate, or even lose continence. The convulsion will usually last for a few minutes and then be followed by a period of drowsiness, confusion, headache, and sleep. When the patients wake up, they may complain of lethargy and muscle aching and notice injuries that they have sustained during the convulsion. For some it can take many hours to recover fully from a tonic–clonic seizure.

Other types of generalized seizures include absence seizures, myoclonic seizures, and atonic and tonic seizures. Absence seizures are a much rarer form of generalized seizures that occur almost exclusively in childhood and early adolescence. The absence may occur many times per day with a duration of up to 15 seconds. The child stares vacantly, the eyes may blink, and excessive swallowing or flopping of the head may occur. These attacks can go unrecognized and only come to light when a child's school performance deteriorates. Atonic and tonic seizures are very rare, accounting for only 1% of the epileptic attacks seen in the general population, but are significant because they may be associated with severe secondary injury. Atonic seizures, or 'drop attacks,' involve a sudden loss of general muscle tone and the patient will fall to the ground. There are no convulsive movements and recovery is usually very rapid. In tonic seizures, patients experience a sudden muscular contraction associated with immediate loss of consciousness and will often fall backwards to the ground. Tonic attacks occur frequently as tonic–clonic episodes in children, but are rare in adults.

Myoclonic seizures are sudden, brief muscle contractions. They often occur in the morning and are occasionally associated with tonic–clonic seizures. Myoclonus is usually termed an epileptic event if it occurs in the context of a seizure disorder without evidence of other brain damage. Other types of myoclonus may occur in the context of progressive and often serious neurological or metabolic disorders.

Where there are inadequate data to classify a seizure type within the sub-categories mentioned above, epilepsy is described as 'unclassified.'

In addition to classifying seizures by type, the International League Against Epilepsy also offers a classification system that groups a number of distinct epileptic syndromes together. This 'syndromic' classification system is based on the observation that, in many patients, a specific constellation of symptoms, signs, and pathologies may often occur together, allowing a doctor to predict likely responses to treatment and even long-term prognosis.

Diagnosis

When doctors are faced with a patient who may have epilepsy, they adopt an approach that is common to the diagnosis of any medical condition. First, a careful history of the presenting complaint is taken and relevant details about the patient's health, medications, and family's health are recorded. In addition, factors in a patient's social life may be pertinent, such as exposure to drugs or alcohol, or an occupation in which head injury may have occurred in the past.

After taking a 'history' from the patient, the doctor will then proceed to perform a physical examination. This examination aims to identify any abnormal medical or neurological 'signs,' which may help to explain a patient's symptoms and support a diagnosis. In many cases of epilepsy, no abnormal signs are discovered on examination, but in others, evidence of disease may be present that make a particular cause for epilepsy more likely. For example, an elderly person developing epilepsy for the first time may have high blood pressure and peripheral vascular disease (circulatory problems) – signs that make atherosclerosis and stroke-related epilepsy more likely.

In most cases of epilepsy, investigations are performed to support the findings of the history and examination. Although several nonspecific tests are performed, which indicate a patient's general health, the mainstays of neurological investigation in epilepsy are the EEG and neuroimaging. Despite recent advances in the technology of these investigations, it is important to realize their limitations. Neither can absolutely refute the possibility that a patient has epilepsy, and many patients with epilepsy have no abnormalities on either their EEG or neuroimaging.

A routine EEG uses monitoring electrodes placed over the scalp of the patient which measure electrical activity present in the brain. Variations of EEG include concomitantly stimulating patients with flashing lights or asking them to perform various physiological maneuvers such as hyperventilating or sleeping. Recordings can be performed over many hours or even days in order to capture the electrical events that are associated with a seizure, and patients may also be video recorded during such prolonged recordings. More specialized EEG monitoring involves surgical insertion of 'deep' electrodes in areas such as the subdural space or even further into the cerebrum.

Although EEG is usually extremely useful in the diagnosis and classification of epilepsy, difficulties arise when recordings are made between seizures (interictally). Approximately 35% of patients with epilepsy show interictal activity indicative of epilepsy in all routine waking recordings, 15% do not show interictal epileptiform abnormalities even after multiple EEGs, and the remainder (50–55%) show epileptiform activity in some but not all recordings. To complicate matters further, a small proportion of people who do not have epilepsy (about 1%) have abnormalities consistent with epilepsy on their EEGs.

Neuroimaging is very different from EEG and involves the use of various techniques to image the brain. These techniques include scans, which examine the structure of the brain, for example computed tomography (CT) and magnetic resonance imaging (MRI), and also techniques which observe the brain's function, such as single-photon emission computed tomography (SPECT) and positron emission tomography (PET). Ideally, adult patients with epilepsy should undergo an MRI scan, which allows a careful examination of the structure of the brain. CT scans achieve a similar result, but involve the use of ionizing radiation and in most cases are unable to match the high resolution and quality achieved by MRI. In many cases, MRI allows patients to be given a very precise diagnosis and a clearer description of the cause of their epilepsy. This information can be invaluable when counselling patients about the prognosis or 'heritability' of their disease.

The technology used in neuroimaging is progressing rapidly. New techniques such as SPECT, PET, and functional MRI are increasingly able to examine the functioning of patients' brains without the need to perform invasive surgical techniques. As these technologies advance, it is likely that further insights into the causes of abnormal central nervous system functioning that is associated with epilepsy will become apparent. Classifications and diagnostic labels based on epilepsy syndromes will become less meaningful than those based on a detailed understanding of an individual's genetics and observed pathologies.

Conclusion

Epidemiological studies demonstrate that epilepsy is very common and affects men and women throughout the world. People who develop epilepsy are often surprised to discover that many individuals of both sexes and all ages suffer from their condition. Epilepsy is an extraordinarily varied condition, and the large numbers of different causes associated with it reflect this. Some of these causes have a genetic basis, but most are likely to result from an interaction between a genetic propensity toward epilepsy and pathologies resulting from environmental factors.

This variety in epilepsy is clearly demonstrated by the large number of classification systems and terminology used to describe epilepsy. Two very useful systems of classification have been offered by the International League Against Epilepsy, but they still only describe epilepsy in terms of its symptoms rather than its causes. Recent advances in technology, in particular in the field of neuroimaging, are transforming the way doctors look at epilepsy and it is likely that, in the near future, breakthroughs in the understanding of the causes and pathologies associated with epilepsy will occur.

SELECTED REFERENCES

Duncan JS, Shorvon SD, Fish DR, eds. *Clinical epilepsy.* Churchill Livingstone, London, 1995.

Sander JWAS, Hart YM. *Epilepsy, questions and answers.* Merit Publishing International, Basingstoke, UK, 1997.

Shorvon SD, Fish D, Thomas D, eds. *The treatment of epilepsy.* Blackwell Science, Oxford, 1996.

7

Antiepileptic drugs and other treatments for epilepsy

Jacqueline A. French

The mainstay of epilepsy treatment is medication. Fortunately, because of a great deal of research in antiepileptic therapy, we now have twice as many antiepileptic drugs available as we did 10 years ago. This is exciting news for people with epilepsy and for their health-care providers. However, it means that antiepileptic drug choice is more complicated. The health-care provider considers seizure type, possible side effects, dosing schedule, safety, and cost in selecting a medication for each individual.

Dr Jacqueline French is an Associate Professor of Neurology at the University of Pennsylvania. She has been involved in the trials leading to the release of all of the new antiepileptic medications, and writes about this topic as well as lecturing to neurologists all over the world.

This chapter provides a comprehensive and comprehensible review of the major antiepileptic drugs, which will be of interest to anyone taking this type of medication. More information about antiepileptic drugs can be found on the Epilepsy Foundation's website at www.epilepsyfoundation.org.

MJM

Once epilepsy is diagnosed, the next step is to decide whether treatment is indicated and, if it is, the best treatment choice. The decision to start medication implies that the benefits to be gained (eliminating or reducing seizure activity) outweigh the potential risks (side effects) and inconvenience. By deciding to take medication, a patient enters into a partnership with her physician.

Open lines of communication are critical. The physician must inform the patient, in the clearest way possible, about the risks and side effects, how to take the medicine, and what to do if there is a problem. The patient must work to follow the prescribed treatment, but she also must be forthcoming with her physician if, for whatever reason, the medication has been taken in a way other than prescribed. Also, the patient must inform her doctor if she experiences any distressing side effects while taking the medication. Frequently, adjusting the medication, or even changing to a new medicine, will solve the problem.

Box 7.1

The patient should never take for granted that feeling bad is 'necessary' to get seizures under control.

How antiepileptic drugs work

The way an antiepileptic drug (AED) works is called its mechanism of action. The available AEDs have many different mechanisms of action. Some (phenytoin, carbamazepine, phenobarbital) work, at least in part, by stabilizing nerve membranes, making it harder for them to fire abnormally and chaotically, as happens during a seizure. Others (valproate, phenobarbital) work partly by increasing inhibition in the brain, thereby 'throwing water on the fire' of epileptic seizures. Newer medications (felbatol, topiramate) may, in addition to other mechanisms, reduce excitatory discharges. Most AEDs are discovered 'by accident.' Compounds are created, and tested in animal models that are meant to mimic human epilepsy. If the compounds raise the seizure threshold, they will be tested further in animals and, eventually, if found safe, may undergo testing in humans. Recently, several AEDs have been developed to have a specific action in the brain. These are called 'designer drugs.' They are the only drugs for which the mechanism of action is certain. Examples of 'designer drugs' are vigabatrin (Sabril, not approved for the US market) and tiagabine (Gabitril, approved but not often prescribed in the USA due to its side effects). Sabril works by preventing a messenger (gamma-aminobutyric acid, GABA) in the brain that inhibits seizures from being broken down. With more of this messenger around, seizures are less likely to occur. Tiagabine also increases the amount of GABA in the brain, but does it by a different mechanism.

Choosing the proper antiepileptic drug

Most people who develop epilepsy think that choosing the right drug to control the seizures should be fairly straightforward. Unfortunately, this is not always the case. To determine which drug is best, the doctor must first classify what types of seizures a person is experiencing. This is usually done by taking a history, and looking at an electroencephalogram (EEG). Once the classification has been determined, there may be many appropriate drugs (Table 7.1).

Recently, many new drugs have been approved. The good news is that there are many more drugs to choose from to select a treatment strategy that is right for the individual patient. However, it is impossible in most cases to determine in advance which drug will be the most effective. This was proven in a study that was performed in the 1980s. In this study, called the Veteran's Administration Cooperative Study, hundreds of patients with the same type of seizures were randomized to one of four drugs – carbamazepine, phenytoin, phenobarbital, and mysoline. The researchers found that the first drug could control seizures about half the time. Those who did not respond to the first drug were randomly assigned to one of the other three. Again, about half gained control of their seizures. The researchers tried to determine anything particular about the patients who were controlled by one drug as opposed to another. Unfortunately, nothing was uncovered.

What this study means for patients with epilepsy is that the very first drug they try might not work and, if it does not, a second or a third drug might. This can be very frustrating, as patients are cycled from drug to drug, but it may be the only way to control seizures. There are many dramatic examples of patients who were having very frequent seizures on the first several drugs that they tried, who finally found the right drug for them, with complete control of seizures.

Because each patient is different and his or her seizures are different, the right dose of medication that will be needed to control seizures without causing side effects must be individually determined. The doctor initially prescribes a standard amount of medicine, frequently based on the patient's body weight. The dose will then be adjusted up or down, depending on any side effects and whether seizures are controlled. If the patient is not having side effects, and all seizures are not controlled, the doctor will gradually

Table 7.1. Seizures and medications for treatment

Seizure types	Useful medications
Partial seizures Simple partial Complex partial Secondary generalized tonic–clonic	Standard: phenytoin, carbamazepine *Newer*: gabapentin, topiramate, lamotrigine, tiagabine, oxcarbazepine, felbamate, levetiracetam
Generalized seizures Absence Myoclonic Generalized tonic–clonic Atonic Tonic	Standard: valproate, ethosuximide (for absence only) *Newer*: lamotrigine, felbamate, topiramate

increase the dose, as a higher amount frequently controls seizures more effectively. Patients going through this will often comment, 'If I tell my doctor I've had a seizure, all he/she does is increase my medicine!' Although the process of finding the right dose of medication can be frustrating, what the doctor is looking for is the exact dose that will control the seizures without producing over-medication. If a medication increase causes side effects, it is time to try a different drug.

The meaning of drug levels

Patients will often hear their physician talk about 'drug levels.' This refers to the fact that only a portion of an ingested drug will enter the bloodstream; the amount of drugs in the blood at any time is called the blood level. Some of the drug may not be absorbed by the intestines, and will be eliminated in the stool. Another portion of the drug may be rapidly changed (metabolized)

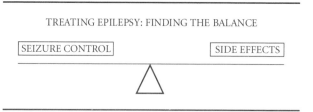

Figure 7.1   Treating epilepsy: finding the balance

by the liver to a substance (metabolite) that is not effective in controlling seizures. Some may leave the body through the kidneys. The amount of drug found in the blood is the only part that can go to the brain and thus have an effect. For most drugs, the effect in the brain is very short lived, and will wax and wane in accordance with the blood level. The blood level does more than just predict the effectiveness of a medication at any time. It may also correlate with side effects. That is, if the blood level dips too low, there may be seizure breakthroughs, whereas if it climbs too high, there may be side effects (Fig. 7.1). Ideally, once the blood level has been found that will control seizures without side effects, it will always stay within a small range, with few peaks and valleys. This is called the therapeutic level. The half-life of a drug (the time until half of the initial amount is eliminated from the body) will determine how often a drug must be taken to keep the blood level within the therapeutic range.

Side effects

A drug's effectiveness is determined by its ability to control seizures. Unfortunately, the drug, by its actions on the body or brain, may cause unwanted side effects as well. There are several types of side effects, but the most common are dose-related side effects. These are problems that may occur when the blood level of a drug gets too high (toxic level). Dose-related side effects may include fatigue, dizziness, lack of coordination, or double vision. Every person has a different threshold at which side effects will appear. Many laboratories, when reporting blood levels to the doctor, will give the doctor a 'therapeutic range.' For example, the therapeutic range for phenytoin is between 10 and 20 μg/ml. This range is based on a population average, and will not be appropriate for all people. Some people will experience side effects with a level below 10 μg/ml, whereas others will have no side effects at levels above 20 μg/ml. Always tell the doctor how you feel and do not accept the 'explanation' that it is not possible for you to have side effects as your drug level is within the therapeutic range.

In addition to dose-related side effects, there may be effects of the medication that are unrelated to the dose and occur in some, but not all, people who take the drug. These are called idiosyncratic (unexpected) side effects. Idiosyncratic side effects might include weight gain or weight loss, tiredness, mental confusion, or depression. If an idiosyncratic side effect occurs, and is affecting the person's quality of life, the drug will probably have to be stopped.

The most feared side effects are those that can cause serious illness. Many people are under the impression that these kinds of problems are more likely if the level is too high or if the drug has been taken for many years. In fact, serious side effects are usually a kind of idiosyncratic reaction, which is unpredictable and not dose-related. These reactions are much more likely to occur early in therapy, and become very rare after the first year. Serious idiosyncratic reactions associated with some AEDs include liver failure, pancreatitis, and fatal blood disorders. It should be stressed that these problems are typically very rare, usually occurring in fewer than 1/100 000 people.

Drug effects specific to women

There has never been a proven difference in AED effects between men and women, although dosages may differ due to differences in body weight. Side effects are also similar in both sexes, but there are certain side effects that may be more troublesome to one sex than to the other. One of these is weight change. Some antiepileptic medications may cause weight gain. This side effect is always idiosyncratic and usually occurs in about one-third of patients. The most profound weight gain is seen in patients taking valproate, who may gain up to 30 lb (13.6 kg). Other drugs, such as carbamazepine and gabapentin, also cause weight gain, but rarely more than 15 lb (6.8 kg). Other drugs, notably felbamate and topiramate, can cause weight loss. The cause of the weight change is unknown, but it is most likely to be due to alterations in basal metabolism. Diet and exercise can help, and the weight usually returns to baseline if the drug is discontinued. Phenytoin, in particular, can cause some cosmetic side effects that are troublesome to women. These include excessive hair growth, including on the face, and coarsening of facial features. These effects do not occur in everyone and are usually the result of long-term use. Because of these effects, many doctors do not prescribe phenytoin to young women.

Some AEDs, including phenytoin, carbamazepine, tiagabine, topiramate, phenobarbital, and mysoline, are metabolized through the liver and speed up the elimination of other substances that are metabolized in the liver. Such drugs are called hepatic enzyme inducers. Some hormones critical to sexual function are metabolized in the liver and levels of these hormonal substances may be reduced by the AEDs listed above. The degree to which this affects human sexual function is controversial. It is also possible that AEDs may affect the pituitary gland directly. Because the pituitary gland regulates hormones, this may also affect sexual function. Patients who take AEDs may notice a reduction in sexual desire or a change in their menstrual cycles.

Oral contraceptives (birth control pills) are also metabolized through the liver and are affected by the presence of enzyme-inducing AEDs. The introduction of such a drug might cause breakthrough bleeding or reduce the contraceptive pill's effectiveness. Therefore, all women taking an enzyme-inducing AED should be on a form of oral contraceptive that contains a higher dose of estrogen (50 μg) or use a barrier method to prevent pregnancy.

Vitamin D, which is also metabolized through the liver, is essential to the body's ability to absorb calcium and build healthy bones. Some patients taking hepatic enzyme-inducing antiepileptic medication have low calcium levels, or osteomalacia. Although osteoporosis has not been definitively linked to long-term AED therapy, it is reasonable for women with epilepsy to take calcium supplements and to discuss with their doctors the need for vitamin D supplementation.

Newer antiepileptic drugs

Several new AEDs have recently been approved by the Food and Drug Administration. These include gabapentin, lamotrigine, topiramate, tiagabine, levetiracetam, and oxcarbazepine. Just like the older drugs, they can be beneficial, but may cause side effects, both dose-related and idiosyncratic.

They are not necessarily better or worse than the established drugs. They do, however, have different mechanisms of action and side-effect profiles. Therefore, they offer potential benefit to people who either have not gained control of their seizures or have had side effects on other drugs they have tried.

Other therapies

Although AEDs are the primary therapeutic modality for epilepsy, and will almost always be tried first, there are other therapeutic options. Some people whose seizures cannot be controlled by AEDs may be candidates for epilepsy surgery.

The epilepsy in about two-thirds of adults is due to a localized area of abnormal brain tissue. This abnormality may consist of a scar from a head injury or infection, a tumor, or an abnormal blood vessel. Sometimes, these abnormalities may show up on a computerized tomography (CT) scan or magnetic resonance imaging (MRI), but sometimes they are microscopic. An EEG may identify the abnormal area because it is electrically excitable. After a comprehensive evaluation, a physician will be able to tell with a good degree of certainty whether seizures are coming from a localized area. In such cases, it may be possible to remove the abnormal area surgically and to eliminate seizures entirely.

The success of this approach will depend on two factors. The first factor is the physician's ability to determine accurately the areas of seizure origin. The second is the possibility of safely removing the affected area without causing any deficits in function. Several tests will assist in this localization of the seizure focus, including MRI, neuropsychological testing (testing of memory and language) positron emission tomography (PET), or single-photon emission computed tomography (SPECT) scan (functional images of the brain) and recording of typical seizures, usually during an inpatient hospital stay. Localization can usually be determined after these tests, but, if not, a neurosurgical procedure to implant EEG electrodes into the areas of the brain where the seizures are thought to originate may be necessary. Once the localization is assured and it has been determined that it is safe to remove the area, surgery can be performed. The most common surgery is called a temporal lobectomy. An evaluation for epilepsy surgery requires the combined efforts of neurologists, neurosurgeons, neuropsychologists, neuroradiologists, and highly skilled EEG technologists. This is best done at a center with staff who have a great deal of experience, most of which are at universities.

People respond very differently to the concept of having surgery. Some see it as a way finally to 'get rid of their problem' once and for all, and to not have to deal with it for the rest of their lives. For these people, the inconvenience, risk, and pain of surgery seem a small price to pay for this enormous benefit. Others are much more fearful of undergoing major surgery that could have potentially irreversible consequences. Epilepsy surgery is not right for everyone, but when appropriate candidates are chosen, and the operation is performed at comprehensive epilepsy center with neurosurgeons experienced in epilepsy surgery, the results can be highly favorable.

A newer technique recently approved for epilepsy treatment is the vagal nerve stimulator. This device is implanted in the chest, much like a pacemaker, with a wire leading to a large nerve in the neck called the vagal nerve. The device sends electrical impulses to the nerve. No one knows why this reduces seizure frequency, but several large studies have convincingly demonstrated its effectiveness. The vagal nerve stimulator will only produce a significant seizure reduction in a proportion of patients who try it, and it is unlikely to make a patient seizure free. However, it does not cause central nervous system side effects, as most AEDs do. For the most part, its use has been limited to those people whose seizures have not been controlled by medication.

Conclusion

Simply put, the AED that controls your seizures with the least side effects is the right AED for you. Keeping an open line of communication with your physician will allow you to work as a 'therapeutic team' and will increase the likelihood that you will find the ideal therapy in the shortest time possible.

SELECTED REFERENCES

Brodie MJ, Dichter MA. Antiepileptic drugs. *N Engl J Med* 1996; 334(3):168–75.
Cramer JA, Mattson RH, Scheyer RD, French J. Review of new antiepileptic drugs. *Epilepsia* 1998; 39(2):233–4.
Dichter MA, Brodie MJ. New antiepileptic drugs. *N Engl J Med* 1996; 334(24):1583–90.
Schachter SC. Antiepileptic drug therapy: general treatment principles and applications for special patient populations. *Epilepsia* 1999; 40(Suppl. 9):S20–5.

8

Epilepsy in children and adolescents

Patricia Crumrine

Dr Patricia Crumrine is Professor of Pediatric Neurology at the University of Pittsburgh. She is a specialist in childhood epilepsy and a former member of the Epilepsy Foundation's Professional Advisory Board.

In this chapter she deals with epilepsy in girls and young women, reviewing the common epilepsy syndromes, treatment challenges, and educational and social concerns.

MJM

Seizures

Approximately 3.5% of all children will have experienced at least one seizure by the age of 15 years. However, only about 1% of children will develop epilepsy or recurrent seizures. Epilepsy arises most frequently during the first year of life. Its incidence (how many people develop the condition) remains high throughout childhood and adolescence and is higher in boys than in girls under the age of 10. Over the age of 10 years, there is not a significant difference between the frequency of development of epilepsy in boys and girls.

The cause of epilepsy is identifiable in only about 24% of childhood cases and is usually developmental. The medical evaluation may include an analysis of the blood cell count, hemoglobin, sugar, calcium, sodium, potassium, as well as other blood tests. The physician may also order an electroencephalogram (EEG), which is a test recording the electrical activity of brain cells. This test may predict the potential of having another seizure. Another possible test is a brain image, usually a magnetic resonance image (MRI) scan. The type of tests ordered depends on the type of seizure, the neurological history and examination, and the results of the EEG.

> **Box 8.1**
>
> *Seizure*   An abnormal electrical discharge of neurons in the brain.
> *Epilepsy*   A chronic disorder in which the main symptom is recurrent
>   seizures that are usually unprovoked and unpredictable.
> **Syndromes**
> *Primary generalized epilepsy* (PGE)   Seizures that affect several parts of the
>   brain and spread to both sides of the brain.
> *Localized related epilepsy* (LRE) Seizures that occur in only an isolated part
>   of the brain, otherwise known as partial seizures.

Following the evaluations, the doctor decides whether there is a need to
take an antiepileptic drug (AED) to prevent further seizures. There are certain
types of seizures that occur only once or infrequently; these seizure types may
not require medicine. If an AED is indicated, your doctor will discuss with
you the type of AED, its frequency of administration, possible side effects,
and the duration of the treatment.

Epileptic syndromes

Some seizure disorders can be grouped together as an epilepsy syndrome.
An epilepsy syndrome is characterized by similar types of seizures, a similar cause, response to medication, and similar findings on EEG and MRI.
It is important to identify whether an individual has a particular epilepsy
syndrome because some of these have a very specific outcome.

Childhood absence epilepsy

Typically, these seizures begin around 7 years of age, but often appear earlier.
They consist of a brief loss of awareness and responsiveness that lasts between
5 and 15 seconds, rarely more than 30 seconds. There may be associated
automatisms, with the seizure consisting of movements of the lips and hands,
and/or fumbling with objects. There is no recall for what happens during the
seizure. These seizures can occur frequently during the day. Therefore, they
may interfere with a child's learning in school. These seizures may also
occur when the child hyperventilates (breathes deeply) or with flashing lights.

This seizure disorder is believed to be genetic or inherited. Up to 44% of first-degree (immediate) relatives may have abnormal EEGs, with a characteristic pattern of generalized 3 per second spike/wave complexes, which is present with or without a seizure. Generalized tonic–clonic seizures may precede or follow the onset of absence seizures. A good long-term outcome can be predicted for most children with this epilepsy syndrome, particularly if there is early onset of absence seizures (4–9 years), normal intelligence, and absence of generalized tonic–clonic seizures. Seventy percent to 80% of children with this type of epilepsy have resolution of their seizures by 10 years of age.

Benign focal epilepsy of childhood with centro-temporal spikes (rolandic seizures)

This is the most common epilepsy syndrome presenting in childhood. It accounts for about 15% of all epilepsies presenting before 15 years of age. It typically begins between 3 and 10 years of age. The most common type of seizure is partial, with movements involving the face, mouth, and occasionally the arms. These seizures frequently occur during sleep or in the early morning hours after wakening. Nighttime seizures usually generalize (become tonic–clonic). Often, seizures are infrequent; some children will only have a single seizure. This is another epileptic syndrome in which genetics play a significant role. Many siblings and first-degree relatives have a history of seizures and febrile convulsions and have EEG abnormalities similar to those seen in the patient. EEG features consist of sharp waves and/or spikes in the centro-temporal (rolandic) area. These occur independently over the two hemispheres of the brain and increase in number with sleep.

This epilepsy syndrome may not require treatment with an AED. When the seizures are infrequent, one option is not to treat. For children who have frequent nocturnal or daytime seizures, treatment with an AED is effective. For those with only nocturnal events, a single nighttime dose of an AED may be helpful. Effective AEDs for this syndrome include those that control the partial seizures: carbamazepine, phenytoin, and phenobarbital. Newer antiepileptics such as gabapentin, lamotrigine, and topiramate may also be effective, although there have not been extensive trials in benign focal epilepsy of childhood (BFEC) using these. A trial of gabapentin for BFEC is currently in progress. Most seizures cease during the mid-adolescent years. Follow-up studies indicate that these seizures do not recur in later life. The EEG pattern disappears later than the clinical seizures.

Benign occipital epilepsy

This is another syndrome that begins during the childhood years, usually around 6–7 years of age. Seizures typically begin with visual symptoms such as brief loss of vision, visual hallucinations characterized by sensations of light or colored discs, or formed visual hallucinations. These visual symptoms may be associated with motor or sensory changes involving one side of the body. Many patients have very severe headaches after a seizure with nausea and/or vomiting. These symptoms may resemble those of migraine headaches.

EEG features are characteristic, showing occipital spike and wave discharges that are often bilateral and disappear when the eyes are opened. The background of the EEG is otherwise normal and appropriate for age. This entity also resolves with age, usually by late adolescence. The treatment options with AEDs are similar to those for BFEC.

Some syndromes with onset during the childhood years do not have a good outcome. Seizures persist once they start and the children often have problems with learning. These syndromes include Lennox–Gastaut syndrome, Landau–Kleffner syndrome (epileptic aphasia), and Rasmussen's encephalitis.

Epileptic syndromes of adolescence

The epileptic syndromes that present in adolescence are juvenile absence epilepsy, juvenile myoclonic epilepsy (JME), and generalized tonic–clonic seizures on awakening. There is considerable overlap of these syndromes. The debate concerns whether they represent distinct syndromes or a spectrum of generalized epilepsy. They are discussed as separate syndromes here. Seizures appearing in adolescence often persist into adult years and are not as responsive to AEDs as those with an earlier onset.

Juvenile absence epilepsy

This syndrome differs from typical childhood absence epilepsy, with a later age of onset. Seizures begin around 9–10 years of age with spells that are shorter and less frequent than those seen in earlier childhood. These may cluster in the morning hours on wakening. More children have associated myoclonic and generalized tonic–clonic seizures with this syndrome than with typical childhood absence epilepsy. The EEG may show a typical 3-Hz generalized spike and wave pattern, but is often faster, at 4–5 Hz. Sodium valproate (VPA) is a very effective AED for juvenile absence epilepsy. Ethosuximide alone is effective when generalized tonic–clonic seizures or myoclonic seizures are not present. Clonazepam is another option for this syndrome, but has a greater incidence of sedation and cognitive effects.

Juvenile myoclonic epilepsy

This epilepsy typically appears at 12–18 years of age. It is a common epilepsy syndrome, appearing in 3–11% of all patients with epilepsy. Clinical features consist of brief, myoclonic jerks of the head, shoulders, and arms on wakening. The affected teenager often appears clumsy, dropping objects from her hands or spilling food. These myoclonic jerks may continue for months or longer before there is a generalized tonic–clonic seizure. Absence seizures occur about 15% of the time.

The EEG shows very fast spikes in association with the myoclonic jerks; 3-Hz spike and wave complexes may also occur. These children are otherwise normal and perform well in school. The clinical history and EEG patterns are sufficient for establishing a diagnosis. Imaging with MRI is usually not necessary. VPA is very effective and controls both the myoclonic and generalized tonic–clonic seizures in most patients. Newer medication may also be effective. Although most people respond very well to valproate, there is about a 95% recurrence rate of seizures if AEDs are withdrawn. Thus, the adolescent will need to continue medication indefinitely.

There is a strong genetic history for this disorder and family histories are usually positive for various types of epilepsy. In some families there is a link of the JME gene to the short arm of chromosome six. There is some suggestion that there may be more than one gene involved.

Generalized tonic–clonic seizures on awakening

Presentation of this syndrome is usually in the mid-teen years, but may appear as early as 8–9 years of age. The syndrome occurs more frequently in females, often with the onset of menarche. Seizures occur within a short period after awakening in the morning, during sleep, and sometimes during periods of relaxation. Precipitating factors include sleep deprivation and flashing lights as from strobe lights, video games, and driving with sun streaming through trees; alcohol ingestion may also play a role.

Many people with generalized tonic–clonic seizures on awakening may also have a history of myoclonic jerks that may precede the onset of the generalized seizures by 1–3 years. Absence seizures are also common. Interictal EEGs (i.e., those done between seizures) may be normal or show generalized polyspike and wave patterns. EEG abnormalities often appear with hyperventilation or intermittent photic stimulation.

Treatment includes the AEDs used for the generalized epilepsies: VPA, benzodiazepines, and lamotrigine. Some young women with this epilepsy syndrome have increased seizures preceding the onset of their menses. For this group, treatment with hormones may be beneficial.

Treatment decisions

Decisions about treating seizures in children and adolescents involve considerations of when to treat, how long to treat, selection of the best medications to use, supplementation with vitamins, and compliance with the treatment plan. For the younger child, these decisions are usually made by the physician and the parents/caretaker. The adolescent should be an active participant in the discussions and decisions. Children and teenagers should understand potential dose-related side effects so that they can relate these to parents if they occur. The physician should ask the child about reasonable dosing times for AEDs related to her school and activity schedules. Children and teenagers should be encouraged to ask questions of the health-care team during office visits.

Antiepileptic drug interactions

Knowledge of possible drug interactions is important, for the physician, the caretakers, and the girl with epilepsy. The use of other medicines or of more than one seizure drug may change the effectiveness of the existing antiepileptic drug and/or the added medication. Antiepileptic drugs that are attached to proteins in the body (protein bound) are most likely to change when another protein-bound drug is added. One example is phenytoin, the level of which may decrease when VPA is added. Many antiepileptic drugs activate liver enzymes that break down the AED, as well as other medications.

Some children have frequent respiratory infections and often require antibiotics, some of which influence the metabolism of the AEDs. For example, erythromycin and isoniazid increase the concentration of carbamazepine and may lead to toxicity. Phenobarbital and phenytoin decrease chloramphenicol levels. Chloramphenicol may increase phenytoin levels. Rifampin (used to treat tuberculosis) decreases phenytoin levels.

Enzyme-inducing AEDs such as carbamazepine, phenobarbital, phenytoin, and primidone decrease the effectiveness of oral contraceptive hormones, resulting in contraceptive failure. Other forms of contraception such as Norplant, a long-acting progesterone-only system, is not as effective in the presence of enzyme-inducing AEDs. It is not known what effect enzyme-inducing AEDs have on Depo-Provera. It appears that felbamate, gabapentin, lamotrigine, and valproate do not decrease the level of oral contraceptive hormones and may not result in contraceptive failure. Because some young women use oral contraceptives to regulate their menstrual periods, knowledge of these drug interactions is extremely important.

Compliance with medication

AED side effects are common at all ages. If the child or adoloscent is aware of the possible side effects, she will be able to report them and her medication dosage can be adjusted. This will improve compliance. Adolescence is a time when active school and extracurricular schedules make adhering to a frequent medication schedule difficult. It is also a time when there is a move for independence and rebellion to authority over issues such as the administration of daily medications. A simple dosing schedule improves compliance and AED levels. Discussing her schedule with the adolescent and the times at which it is easier for her to take medicine often improves compliance. Changing from multiple doses per day to dosing twice a day or once a day, using sustained release forms of AEDs or AEDs with long half-lives, is also a helpful alternative.

Alternative therapies

For children whose seizures are not controlled with AEDs, there are some alternative therapies. One of these is the use of a high-fat (ketogenic) diet that restricts carbohydrates, proteins, and fluids. It is most effective in the preschool child with myoclonic/astatic seizures, i.e., drop attacks involving loss of muscle tone that causes the child to drop to the floor and begin jerking motions. Studies of the efficacy of the ketogenic diet reveal that about 30% of children obtain seizure control, another 30% achieve approximately 50% reduction in their seizures, and 40% have no significant reduction in their seizures. There has not been much experience using the ketogenic diet for adolescents. If a family is considering this diet for a teenager attending regular school, she should be an active participant in the discussion. The adolescent should know what the dietary restrictions will be and what impact this would have on her lifestyle. The diet should not be tried without the adolescent's consent, except if she is unable to make appropriate decisions.

Vitamin supplementation

Some AEDs, for example phenytoin, alter the concentration of vitamin D in the body. Other factors include exposure to sunlight and adequate dietary sources. Women who are unable to go out because of other motor impairments may develop osteomalacia (decreased mineralization of the bone). They may need supplementation with vitamin D, 400 IU daily.

Some AEDs deplete the levels of folic acid. Deficiencies of folic acid may contribute to a higher rate of birth defects in the children of women with epilepsy. Therefore, women of childbearing age (at menarche) should receive low doses of folate (0.4–0.8 mg/day) in the form of a multivitamin tablet or dietary supplements. Higher doses of folate (4 mg/day) should be reserved for women with a history of pregnancies resulting in neural tube defects, or with a family history of such defects.

Educational, behavioral, and social issues

Educational issues

Although the majority of children with epilepsy have normal intelligence and school achievement, some have intellectual and educational disabilities. Children with epilepsy and lower intelligence tend to have developed epilepsy at an early age, have had brain injury or widespread brain dysfunction, have had epilepsy for many years, or refused therapy with multiple antiepileptic drugs. Children and adolescents who have normal cognitive development include those with febrile seizures, childhood absence epilepsy, benign focal epilepsy (rolandic epilepsy) and JME. Better seizure control (fewer seizures) improves learning as assessed by standardized neuropsychological tests.

Behavioral issues

Occassional mood swings and behavioral outbursts are normal for all children, especially for teenagers. However, behavioral problems may be more common in children and adolescents with epilepsy. Behavior problems are more common when seizures are poorly controlled and when multiple AEDs are used. Particular AEDs may be more likely to cause this type of problem. Researchers note a higher incidence of behavioral problems (conduct disturbance and hyperactivity) and depression in children taking phenobarbital. Phenytoin and VPA may also negatively affect behavior. Benzodiazepines often contribute to behavioral problems, with increased irritability and aggression.

Peer issues

A frequently asked question by teenagers is 'Who should I tell, or not tell, that I have epilepsy?' It is very helpful for the child and the adolescent to have at least one 'best friend' who knows about the epilepsy – specifically, what happens when the seizure occurs and how to handle the situation. The parents of good friends should also know about the seizures. As young girls often sleep over at friends' houses, and seizures frequently occur at night or on waking in the morning, the host should know what to do should a seizure occur.

As teenagers spend most of their time away from their parents and home, they should have a confidante who knows about their seizures and medicines. This may be a difficult discussion for the adolescent, who does not want to be different from her peers. A parent or the teenager's doctor can help with the discussion. Inviting the friend to attend the child's doctor visits is a way of providing this information. Telling a boyfriend about seizures is also a very difficult task. Because the teenager often feels insecure about herself and her relationships, she may be hesitant to relay this personal information to a boyfriend. For women who have not had seizures for 6–12 months, relaying this information at the onset of a relationship may not be absolutely necessary. If the relationship becomes long term, the teenager should discuss her epilepsy. For women who have uncontrolled seizures, relating this information in a straightforward way early in the relationship may avoid the difficult task of explaining the seizures after one occurs. If the teenager has a job, she should tell her immediate coworkers about her seizures.

Recreational drugs and alcohol

Adolescence is a time of experimentation. Experimentation with drugs and alcohol may have a significant impact on seizure control, by lowering the seizure threshold or changing the body's metabolism of the antiepileptic drug used to treat the seizures. Parents, caretakers, and the adolescent herself need to be aware of the risks associated with alcohol and some recreational drugs. It is helpful for the young woman with epilepsy to discuss these issues privately with a member of her health-care team.

Driving issues for the adolescent

Sixteen is an exciting year for the adolescent. In the USA, this is the year when she can obtain her driver's permit and license. Knowing that she will need to be seizure free prior to applying for the license often helps to improve compliance for taking AEDs. For the adolescent with uncontrolled epilepsy, this is a difficult time because it represents another limitation of her activities compared to those of her peers. It may impact her social activities and employment potential as well.

Each state has its own set of regulations pertaining to driving. Regulations vary from state to state pertaining to the length of the seizure-free interval needed before a license can be granted. The type of seizure (whether consciousness is impaired) may also be considered. Other variables considered include whether seizures occur only during sleep, during an illness, or during drug or alcohol withdrawal, which may not necessarily develop into epilepsy. The treating physician should become familiar with the state's regulations and begin discussing these with the teenager when she is 13–14 years old. Only six states (California, Delaware, Nevada, New Jersey, Oregon, and Pennsylvania) still have mandatory physician reporting laws that require the treating physician to notify the state's department of motor vehicles that a person has epilepsy.

Discontinuation of antiepileptic drugs

Several epileptic syndromes resolve during the adolescent years. These teenagers may stop their AEDs after a tapering period. Syndromes that may allow medication withdrawal include childhood absence and benign focal epilepsy. For young women whose seizures do not relate to a prior brain insult such as meningitis, encephalitis, trauma, or a stroke, medication withdrawal is possible after seizure control for 2 years. If a person is taking more than one AED, the treating physician should decide which AED to withdraw first. AED withdrawal should always be done with the permission and under the guidance of the treating doctor. It is never wise to withdraw medicine on one's own. The rate of AED taper depends on the type of medicine and the duration of the AED. Some AEDs can be tapered faster than others, for example, one can withdraw ethosuximide and valproate in a short period compared to AEDs such as phenobarbital and the benzodiazepines, which take several weeks to a couple of months to taper and stop. The treating physician should review the risk of seizure recurrence before tapering the medicine. Then the patient and her family should choose the best time to begin the AED taper.

The likelihood that medication can be stopped is highest in those who have been seizure free for 2 or more years, who have a normal neurological examination, normal cognitive function, normal brain imaging, a single seizure type, rapid response to AEDs, onset of seizures after the age of 3–4, infrequent seizures, and no history of atonic, tonic, or complex partial seizures or status epilepticus. If these factors are present, the chances of becoming and remaining seizure free are about 70%. Girls with JME, juvenile absence, and generalized tonic–clonic seizures on awakening have a high rate of recurrence if they withdraw their AEDs. Thus, for this population, AEDs are continued indefinitely. Also, for those adolescents whose seizures begin during their teenage years, there is a higher seizure recurrence rate following the discontinuation of AEDs.

Conclusion

Childhood and adolescence can be particularly challenging times for girls dealing with epilepsy. However, the better educated she is about her epilepsy, combined with open and honest communication with parents and doctors, the more empowered a girl will be. Teachers and school nurses can also play an important role. The more understanding there is about epilepsy, the more accepted any child or teenager with epilepsy will be by her peers. With this foundation, a young woman can be helped to make the transition into a happy and productive adult.

SELECTED REFERENCES

Aicardi J. *Epilepsy in Children.* Raven Press, New York, 1994.

Dodson WE. Pharmacokinetic principles of antiepileptic therapy in children. In *Pediatric Epilepsy: Diagnosis and Therapy,* ed. WE Dodson, JM Pellock. Demos Publications, New York, 1993, 231–40.

Duchowny M, Harvey AS. Pediatric epilepsy syndromes. An update and critical review. *Epilepsia* 1996; 37 (Suppl. 1):S26–40.

Guarino EJ, Morrell MJ. Management of the adolescent with epilepsy: hormones, antiepileptic drugs and reproductive health. *Int Pediatr* 1995; 10 (Suppl. 1):66–71.

Leppick IE. Metabolism of antiepileptic medications: newborn to elderly. *Epilepsia* 1992; 33 (Suppl. 4):32–44.

Mims J. Sexuality and related issues in the preadolescent and adolescent female with epilepsy. *J Neurosci Nurs* 1996; 28(2):102–6.

Morrell MJ. Hormones and epilepsy through the lifetime. *Epilepsia* 1992; 33 (Suppl. 4): S49–S61.

Trimble MR. Behavioral and cognitive issues in childhood epilepsy. In *Pediatric Epilepsy: Diagnosis and Therapy,* ed. WE Dodson, JM Pellock. Demos Publications, New York, 1993, 387–408.

Wildrick D, Parker-Fisher S, Morales A. Quality of life in children with well-controlled epilepsy. *J Neurosci Nurs* 1996; 28(3):192–8.

9

Nonepileptic seizures

Steven C. Schachter

Epileptic seizures are transient events of altered neurological function that occur because of paroxysmal brain electrical activity. Other events of altered neurological function may look very much like seizures, but are not caused by electrical brain activity. Epileptic seizure-like events may be caused by changes in blood pressure, heart rate and rhythm, or by changes in blood sugar. Emotional triggers may also cause transient epileptic seizure-like events. Stress, depression, and anxiety may cause physical symptoms that closely resemble seizures. In fact, it may not be possible for a physician to tell the difference between an emotionally triggered seizure – called a psychogenic seizure – and an epileptic seizure unless an electroencephalogram (EEG) can be recorded during the event. The EEG shows brain electrical activity and will differentiate epileptic and nonepileptic seizures.

Dr Steven Schachter is Associate Professor of Neurology at Harvard Medical School and an epileptologist at Beth Israel Deaconess Medical Center. He is Chair of the Professional Advisory Board of the Epilepsy Foundation.

In this chapter, Dr Schachter deals with nonepileptic seizures, drawing from his knowledge of the field and his own personal experience caring for individuals with this condition. Diagnosis may be difficult, but is especially important in order to ensure that the right kind of treatment is provided.

MJM

What are nonepileptic seizures?

Nonepileptic seizures are behavioral events that look to other people like epileptic seizures or are events that create internal sensations that may also occur in people who have epileptic seizures. When medical professionals use the term epileptic seizures, they are referring to behavioral events caused by abnormal electrical discharges or disruptions in the brain and, in particular, its outer layer, the cortex. These electrical disruptions occur only during epileptic seizures and can generally be detected with a brain wave test – an electroencephalogram (EEG) – if the test is taken *during* such a seizure. By definition, nonepileptic seizures are not caused by electrical disruptions in the brain, yet to observers they may resemble tonic–clonic, absence, or complex partial epileptic seizures.

Even trained medical personnel may have trouble telling the difference between some types of nonepileptic seizures and epileptic seizures just by watching them. It is not surprising, then, that health-care providers often mistake nonepileptic seizures for epileptic seizures. Consequently, nonepileptic seizures in some patients may be inaccurately diagnosed as epileptic seizures and the patients started on antiepileptic drugs (AEDs). However, whereas AEDs are helpful in treating epileptic seizures, they are of no benefit in treating nonepileptic seizures.

Doctors classify nonepileptic seizures into two major types: psychogenic and physiologic. Psychogenic nonepileptic seizures are thought to result from stressful psychological conflicts or major emotional trauma. Physiologic nonepileptic seizures are caused by a sudden change in the blood supply to the brain or in the delivery of sugar or oxygen to the brain. The causes of physiologic nonepileptic seizures include rhythm disturbances of the heart, sudden drops in blood pressure, and very low blood sugar. Primary care physicians often diagnose physiologic nonepileptic seizures as fainting spells, syncope, cardiac arrhythmia, or hypoglycemia.

Psychogenic nonepileptic seizures are more challenging to recognize and diagnose than physiologic nonepileptic seizures; therefore, this chapter focuses on psychogenic nonepileptic seizures, which are referred to simply as nonepileptic seizures.

There are several consequences of mistaking nonepileptic seizures for epileptic seizures. Perhaps the most significant of them is that AEDs will probably be recommended, thus putting the individual at risk for the systemic or cognitive side effects of AEDs without potential benefit. In addition, the diagnosis of epileptic seizures brings with it a societal stigma that adds further unnecessary stress. An accurate diagnosis of nonepileptic seizures is critical to successful treatment and for the patient to be safely taken off AEDs. Sometimes, but not always, there are enough clues when symptoms first develop to suggest the diagnosis of nonepileptic seizures. In those instances, the doctor may order EEG testing (described below) even before prescribing an AED. More typically, months to years of unsuccessful AED therapy elapse, calling into question the diagnosis of epileptic seizures and raising the possibility of nonepileptic seizures.

Nonepileptic seizures are fairly common. Twenty percent of the patients evaluated at epilepsy centers have nonepileptic seizures. Some of these patients also have epileptic seizures. This can make the accurate diagnosis of nonepileptic seizures very difficult, especially in patients with a past history of epilepsy in whom a new seizure type develops.

What causes nonepileptic seizures?

Although doctors do not yet know what causes nonepileptic seizures, it is clear that most affected patients have unresolved stressful psychological problems, often stemming from abuse (sexual and/or physical) in childhood or a major life event such as death or divorce, but the connections between these issues and nonepileptic seizures vary considerably from patient to patient. Not all people with these problems have nonepileptic seizures, not all patients with nonepileptic seizures carry these psychological burdens, and some patients with epileptic seizures have similar psychological difficulties.

The underlying physiology of nonepileptic seizures is not known and there are no tests that prove what is happening in the brain during them – tests can only show what is *not* happening. Therefore, some doctors may give the impression that they believe their patients with nonepileptic seizures are 'faking' their seizures to gain attention. In fact, another term used for psychogenic nonepileptic seizures can convey this same regrettable attitude – pseudoseizure. This terminology is unfortunate, because there is nothing pseudo, false, or fake about nonepileptic seizures to patients who have them. From their perspective, these patients are having real seizures. If these patients are allowed to think that they deliberately cause their seizures, the healing process will probably be impeded. Moreover, the relationship between women and their physicians has a history of an imbalance of power. In the past, many women have been told that their illnesses are 'all in your head' and have been left with no alternatives for treatment. Although psychogenic nonepileptic seizures do not show up on an EEG, they are nonetheless a serious condition and, with proper care, can be treated.

Is there anything in a patient's background that might suggest the diagnosis of nonepileptic seizures? The patient with nonepileptic seizures may have a history of having experienced one or more significant traumatic events, such as sexual or physical abuse. Often, the patient will have repressed these past experiences but may recall them during a session with a supportive mental health professional. Sometimes the abusive act is relived during the nonepileptic seizure, while the patient is unconscious.

The patient's history may offer several other clues that increase the possibility of her having nonepileptic seizures. For example, she may have previously encountered people with epileptic seizures. Perhaps she has a relative with epilepsy, once had a hospital roommate with epilepsy, or witnessed someone having an epileptic seizure at work, in a workshop, or at school. A previous personal history of epileptic seizures also increases the possibility of nonepileptic seizures. This situation is particularly challenging because medication changes should ideally be made only on the basis of a patient's epileptic seizures, not her nonepileptic seizures. EEG monitoring may be necessary to document which seizures are epileptic and which are nonepileptic. Other clues include unsuccessful treatment with AEDs, frequent emergency room visits or hospitalizations for seizures, and a history of psychiatric illness (particularly anxiety, panic attacks, and depression).

How can doctors tell the difference between epileptic seizures and nonepileptic seizures?

Just as with epileptic seizures, the diagnosis of nonepileptic seizures depends on accurate seizure descriptions by the patient and any other people who have observed the seizures. However, the descriptions of nonepileptic seizures may be very similar to those for epileptic seizures. Therefore, the diagnosis may not be suspected until the patient undergoes a prolonged trial of one or more AEDs without gaining control over the seizures.

Although the behaviors that occur during nonepileptic seizures are very similar to those associated with epileptic seizures, they may differ in several respects. For example, whereas epileptic seizures occur whether or not anyone else is present, nonepileptic seizures usually (but not always) happen in front of a witness. Seizure-related injuries, such as broken bones, are more typical of epileptic seizures than of nonepileptic seizures. An absence of significant emotional stress preceding the seizure would argue more for an epileptic seizure.

Nonepileptic seizures that resemble tonic–clonic seizures are the least problematic to differentiate. They usually begin gradually, with motor activity that slowly escalates in intensity, whereas epileptic tonic–clonic seizures begin abruptly. A cry or shriek in the middle of the seizure or at the end is suggestive of an nonepileptic seizure, as are motor movements that come and go, that alternately affect the left and right sides of the body, or that look like sexual behaviors, such as pelvic thrusting. Unusual posturing may also occur during nonepileptic seizures, but facial muscle contractions are uncommon. An apparent convulsive seizure that extends for many minutes, perhaps even to 1 hour or longer, is probably nonepileptic, especially if there is no cyanosis (blue skin coloring) and the patient wakes up immediately after the seizure movements stop. The recovery period (postictal state) that follows a convulsive-appearing nonepileptic seizure is brief, whereas recovery from a tonic–clonic seizure lasts minutes to a couple of hours and is characterized by confusion, headache, exhaustion, and sleep.

Nonepileptic seizures that look like absence or complex partial seizures are more difficult to distinguish from epileptic seizures, and even experts can mistake these for epileptic seizures, and *vice versa*. One clue is the duration: absence seizures usually last less than 15 seconds, and complex partial seizures generally end within 5 minutes. Events that have the behavioral characteristics of these seizure types but last considerably longer should be considered possible nonepileptic seizures. Otherwise, there are few clinical features that allow for the accurate identification of non-convulsive nonepileptic seizures. Even behaviors that appear bizarre may be epileptic. For example, electrical disruptions in the frontal lobes can cause strange movements and vocalizations, minimally affect consciousness, and end without a postictal state. Of all the types of epileptic seizures that are mistaken for nonepileptic seizures, those of frontal lobe origin are probably the most common.

It cannot be overemphasized that these clues are not foolproof. Neither epileptic seizures nor nonepileptic seizures can be unquestionably diagnosed from historical features or aspects of the seizures themselves. EEG monitoring should be obtained when there is sufficient reason to question the diagnosis. Ultimately, the diagnosis of nonepileptic seizures depends on the results of EEG monitoring, because no clues from the patient's history or seizure descriptions are absolutely diagnostic of nonepileptic seizures.

What is the best way to diagnose nonepileptic seizures?

EEG monitoring is the best way to make an accurate diagnosis of nonepileptic seizures. This test involves recording the brain rhythms of the patient for a prolonged period, typically for one or more days, usually in the hospital and while video images of the patient are also being recorded. The goal is to record the EEG during several, if possible, typical seizures. Simultaneously recording the video image of the patient while he or she has a typical seizure allows the family or other observers to verify that the recorded seizure is the same seizure that they have previously witnessed. Sometimes, when necessary, the patient is taken off AEDs. At some centers, patients are encouraged to carry out activities that are likely to bring on their seizures, such as arguing with a family member, or staying up all night. If no seizures occur for several days, the patient's doctor may try to induce a seizure with special provocative tests.

EEG monitoring has four possible outcomes.

1 The EEG may confirm that the patient's seizures are epileptic seizures.
2 The EEG may be suggestive, but not diagnostic, of epileptic seizures. In that situation, so-called invasive electrodes (EEG electrodes that are surgically implanted into the brain) may be recommended if the patient is a candidate for epilepsy surgery. This is usually scheduled for another time.
3 The EEG may not show any abnormality whatsoever before, during, or after the patient's seizure. This finding is very suggestive of nonepileptic seizures, particularly if the patient's seizure appears to be the tonic–clonic type. However, this testing is not infallible and some epileptic seizures are only apparent on the EEG when recorded with invasive electrodes.
4 The patient may not have any typical seizures while in the hospital. In this case, no progress can be made in the diagnostic evaluation, but absence of proof is not proof of absence.

EEG monitoring can be done on an outpatient basis if: (1) the patient has seizures every 1–2 days or has a seizure only in a particular environment outside the hospital, and (2) the patient is closely observed by someone who is willing to write down his or her seizure observations on the log sheet that accompanies the EEG monitoring device. However, if these conditions do not exist, then it is advisable to admit the patient to hospital for video–EEG testing.

EEG monitoring is a highly specialized procedure performed at epilepsy referral centers. It involves a team of professionals: EEG readers, EEG technicians, epilepsy nurses, ward nurses, resident physicians, the attending physician, and computer engineers. It is critical that the quality of the testing is sufficient to accomplish the goals set out when the testing began. A psychiatric evaluation is often part of the diagnostic evaluation, and patients may undergo neuropsychological testing as well.

What is the treatment for nonepileptic seizures and what is the outlook?

Treatment begins when the results of EEG monitoring (including the findings of the provocative tests, if done) are discussed with the patient. It is crucial that a physician with whom the patient has established a trusting relationship presents the results to the patient.

Discussing the test results may require more than one session. The manner and tone with which the doctor conveys the findings to the patient can help or hinder the patient's acceptance of and willingness to enter into treatment. Different doctors have different ways of handling this conversation. My own approach is to describe the EEG results while acknowledging the limitations of EEG testing and the diagnostic process for nonepileptic seizures in general. I then explain that the brain has many systems that work simultaneously – electrical, chemical, hormonal, vascular, and others that scientists have not yet discovered – and that any one of these systems could conceivably become dysfunctional and produce nonepileptic seizures. The electrical system is the only one that we can presently test. Therefore, showing that the patient's seizures are not caused by electrical disturbances does not mean that there is no problem at all; it only means that the electrical system is not the culprit. Unfortunately, despite the wonders of modern medicine, doctors cannot readily measure the other systems during seizures, particularly those affected by psychological stress. However, although doctors cannot prove the underlying cause because of the limitations of current tests, they can help the patient to focus on those sources of stress or other life experiences that trigger the nonepileptic seizures and work with the patient to eliminate those triggers or alleviate their emotional impact. These goals are the foundation of treatment.

The key for the physician is to approach the patient with empathy and understanding. The key for the patient is to be willing to search for and recognize the influence of internal emotional stresses on the genesis of the seizures and to explore these issues once the diagnosis of nonepileptic seizures is established.

Generally, the conclusion that the patient's events are not caused by electrical seizures should be presented as good news. The positive implications are that: (1) AEDs, along with their possible side effects, are not necessary (unless the patient also has other seizures that are electrical), and (2) with supportive care, usually involving psychological help and the passage of time, the events will probably improve. In fact, the prognosis is better than for epileptic seizures, especially when the nonepileptic seizures have only recently begun. Because there is a significant chance of complete recovery, it is important to make the correct diagnosis as early as possible.

To motivate the patient further to enter into a therapeutic relationship with a mental health provider, the physician should help her acknowledge the disabling nature of the seizures and their psychosocial effects on her life. The neurologist will usually suggest that the very best supportive treatment the patient can receive is individual attention from a psychologically oriented professional who is knowledgeable about nonepileptic seizures and experienced in their treatment. Medications may be suggested if depression or anxiety is a significant part of the picture. The neurologist will usually collaborate with the psychiatrist or other mental health professional. Other health-care providers may become involved as well, such as a social worker or nurse specialist.

At many epilepsy centers, a team of professionals, all affiliated with the epilepsy center, manages the treatment of nonepileptic seizures. The goals of therapy are set by the team in conjunction with the patient and generally include restoration of function with reduction in the severity and frequency of the nonepileptic seizures. The outlook is enhanced when every member of the team, including the patient, approaches the therapeutic process with a positive attitude. The importance of having a positive attitude cannot be overstated.

Summary

Nonepileptic seizures, especially those that look like absence or complex partial seizures, are often difficult for physicians to distinguish from epileptic seizures, for two reasons. First, nonepileptic seizures may resemble true epileptic seizures to observers. Second, some patients have both nonepileptic seizures and epileptic seizures. Nonepileptic seizures are of two types: psychogenic and physiologic. The former type is more difficult to diagnose. Physiologic nonepileptic seizures are caused by a sudden change in the blood supply to the brain or in the delivery of sugar or oxygen to the brain, whereas psychogenic nonepileptic seizures are believed to result from stressful psychological conflicts or emotional trauma. The patient's history may offer several clues to psychogenic nonepileptic seizures, but these clues are not definitive. They include a history of sexual or physical abuse, previous exposure to people with epileptic seizures, or a personal history of epileptic seizures. The best way to diagnose psychogenic nonepileptic seizures accurately is by EEG monitoring. If the diagnosis is confirmed, treatment consists of therapy conducted by a mental health counselor who is experienced in the treatment of psychogenic nonepileptic seizures. If indicated, antidepressant or anti-anxiety medications may also be prescribed. A positive outlook on the part of the patient and the health-care team is essential for a good outcome in the diagnosis and treatment of nonepileptic seizures.

SELECTED REFERENCES

Alper K, Devinsky O, Perrine K, Vazquez B, Luciano D. Nonepileptic seizures and childhood sexual and physical abuse. *Neurology* 1993; 43:1950–3.

Chabolla DR, Krahn LE, So EL, Rummans TA. Psychogenic nonepileptic seizures. *Mayo Clin Proc* 1996; 71:493–500.

Rowan AJ. Nonepileptic seizures. In *The Comprehensive Evaluation and Treatment of Epilepsy. A Practical Guide,* ed. SC Schachter, DL Schomer. Academic Press, San Diego, 1997, pp. 173–183.

Rowan AJ, Gates JR, eds. *Non-epileptic seizures.* Butterworth–Heinemann, Boston, 1993.

Schachter SC. *Brainstorms: Epilepsy in Our Words.* Raven Press, New York, 1993.

Shen W, Bowman ES, Markand ON. Presenting the diagnosis of pseudoseizure. *Neurology* 1990; 40:756–9.

Trimble MR. Pseudoseizures. *Neurol Clin* 1966; 4:531–48.

Part III

Hormones and the brain

10

Brain differences

Paula Shear and Rosemary Fama

Dr Paula Shear is a neuropsychologist who has worked with men and women with epilepsy to study brain functioning. Dr Rosemary Fama is a research associate at SRI International. They bring this knowledge and experience to this chapter, in which they review the differences in brain development, organization, and functioning between men and women. For example, whereas men and women have similar intelligence, men tend to be stronger with visual–spatial and mathematical tasks, and women have stronger verbal abilities. These brain differences mean that men and women with epilepsy may be more or less likely to develop particular types of difficulties. These differences are of particular importance as we consider how epilepsy might affect men and women differently, and also as we think about the potential side effects of epilepsy treatments such as medications and surgery.

MJM

This chapter provides an overview of the differences between men and women in terms of brain development, normal cognitive (thinking) skills, and the cognitive difficulties that may result from epilepsy. Although men and women have more similarities than differences in their brain development and brain functioning, a large body of scientific literature supports the presence of small but meaningful differences between their brains. The emphasis of this chapter is on the biology of sex differences in brain functioning, but there are many 'nonbiological' factors that also explain differences in behavior between men and women (Fig. 10.1).

From infancy, boys and girls are socialized differently in our culture. There is often a tendency to encourage 'gender-appropriate' behavior in both children and adults. For example, newborn babies of either sex who are dressed to look like girls are perceived as more delicate and are handled more gently by adults than are the same babies dressed to look like boys. The effects of socialization highlight the fact that the differences between the behaviors of men and women are due to biology *and* culture.

Brain development

At conception, each parent contributes one sex chromosome to his or her child's genetic makeup. Because women have two X chromosomes, the mother can only give an X chromosome to the child; the father can give either an X or Y chromosome. If the baby receives the chromosome combination XX from its parents, it will be genetically female; a baby receiving the chromosome XY combination will be genetically male. With the exception of the difference in a single sex chromosome, early embryos that will develop into boys and girls are otherwise identical. The Y chromosome carries genetic material that causes the embryo to develop testes; in the absence of this material, ovaries develop.

Within the first trimester of a human pregnancy, the male testes begin to produce the sex hormone testosterone, which causes the brain to become 'masculinized' and also causes the male genitals to develop. If testosterone is present during certain critical windows of time during prenatal development, these masculinizing changes will occur and will be permanent. If testosterone is not available or is available at the wrong time during development, these changes will never occur. It is clear that male hormones (androgens) and female hormones (estrogens) that present very early in development drive a complex chain of events that permanently alter the way certain parts of the brain and the body are organized.

Initial research examining the effects of testosterone looked not at changes in the brain itself, but rather at the effects of this hormone on genital development and adult sexual behavior in animals. The majority of these studies involved rats, because the critical period for the hormonal effect in rats is near the time of birth, making research that examines the effects of the hormonal environment easier than if manipulations had to be made while the fetus was still inside the womb. Moreover, in contrast to the wide range of sexual behaviors that humans display, rats have stereotyped male and female sexual behavior. In other words, it is clear when a rat is displaying sex-appropriate sexual behavior, which makes studies of sexual behavior in these animals straightforward.

Early studies showed that when genetically male animals (chromosomes XY) had surgery to remove the testes very early in development (thus depriving them of testosterone), they developed female genitalia. As adults, these rats showed female sexual behavior and the female cycles of hormone production levels similar to the human woman's menstrual cycle. When their testes were removed early in development but they were treated with testosterone within the critical period, they developed normal male sexual anatomy and behavior and male noncyclic hormonal production. Thus, early testosterone exposure in animals is clearly important to normal male sexual development. In contrast, genetically female rats that had their ovaries removed early in development nevertheless showed normal female sexual behavior as adults. If genetically female rats were treated with testosterone during the critical period, however, they showed male sexual behavior as adults. From this series of studies, scientists concluded that female sexual anatomy and behavior are the 'default pattern' that develops in the absence of testosterone, and that adult sexual behavior in the rat is dependent not only on the animal's genetic sex, but also on the hormonal environment that is present during critical periods in early development. It is now known that normal female development is not entirely a default pattern, in that it also requires certain hormones to be present in low doses.

Building on these foundation studies, researchers began to explore whether sex differences extended beyond genital development and sexual behavior. In humans, testosterone binds directly to certain brain receptors, but also can be converted by a chemical process to an estrogen, which in turn acts at specific receptors in brain cells. These steroid hormone receptors are located in many different brain regions, although they have the highest concentrations in regions that are responsible for the control of sexual behavior and hormone regulation. If brain tissue that contains these receptors is placed in culture outside the body and treated with testosterone or with estrogens, the neurons show dramatically enhanced growth. Thus, the early hormonal environment in the body has the potential to cause actual changes in brain structure by altering growth patterns in specific brain regions.

In rats, the difference in size of the hypothalamus (a region of the brain referred to as the 'sexually dimorphic nucleus of the preoptic area'), which regulates hormone cycles and sexual behavior, is so striking that the sex of the animal can be determined reliably on this basis alone. Furthermore, the size of the sexually dimorphic nucleus of the hypothalamus in adult animals is directly related to the amount of testosterone available early in development, leading to the theory that the early hormonal environment directly causes growth in the sexually dimorphic nucleus.

There are other differences in brain structure between men and women. For example, after the differences in head size between men and women are taken into account, women have much larger brain volumes in regions that are related to language functioning and also a thicker corpus callosum, the large bundle of fibers that interconnects the two hemispheres of the brain (Fig. 10.1).

In addition to differences in the size of certain brain structures in men and women, provocative recent studies suggest that their brains may function slightly differently. Sex differences are reported in the amount of blood flow in the brain and in the pattern of glucose metabolism (energy utilization) in different brain regions. Brain changes with age may also be different in men and women. As the brain ages, fluid increases and tissue shrinks. Older men show more pronounced tissue loss in certain brain regions than do older women. These studies suggest that sex differences are an important part of brain development throughout the lifespan. They also explain why brain function is different in men and women.

Cognitive skills in men and women

Cognitive skills refer to 'thinking' in areas such as language, memory, and visual–spatial processing. Despite comparable general intelligence, the performance of cognitive skills is different in healthy men and women (and girls and boys). These cognitive sex differences are seen even in preschool-aged children. On average, males score better than females on visual–spatial and mathematical tasks, whereas females score better on certain verbal tasks. It is important to emphasize that these cognitive sex differences are rather small and have not been confirmed in all studies. In addition, the studies tell us only that large groups of men and women tend to perform differently on certain cognitive tasks. They do not suggest that all men are superior to all women on spatial tasks or that all women are superior to all men on verbal tasks. There are certainly many women who show exceptional spatial and mathematical abilities and many men who show outstanding verbal skills. In addition, sex differences are not evident on all verbal and spatial tasks. In verbal skills,

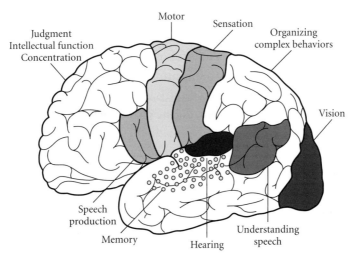

Figure 10.1 Locations of general brain functions.

females tend to outscore males on tasks assessing word fluency, articulation, grammar, reading comprehension, and verbal memory, but males score better than females on tasks of verbal analogies. Similarly with spatial tasks, males outscore females on visual–spatial tasks assessing mental rotation (the ability to mentally rotate figures in space), but no differences are found on spatial perception tasks (the ability to find a figure that is embedded in a more complex figure), and females have been reported to outperform males on visual tasks that require psychomotor speed and accuracy. There is also evidence that men and women often apply different strategies when they approach certain cognitive tasks, and their performance differences may reflect not only raw ability but also the strategy that is employed to solve a particular problem.

Cognitive differences between males and females have received considerable attention in the popular press. One issue that has generated a great deal of discussion is the reported difference between boys and girls on the Scholastic Aptitude Test (SAT), the college entrance exam taken by high-school students, generally during their junior year. The SAT yields two general scores, one verbal and one quantitative. On average, boys score higher on the quantitative part of the exam (by about 50 points). Whether this difference is due to biological (i.e., genetically based differences) or environmental (i.e., socialization, life experiences) factors has been debated. Some authors contend that males and females differ in these ability areas because of innate biological differences, such as differences in brain structure, whereas others believe that the differences reflect how men and women are socialized. For example, boys often receive more encouragement to take and excel in science and mathematics courses than do girls. It is most likely that both biology and experience contribute to many of the cognitive difference between women and men.

Cognitive differences associated with the hormonal environment

It is not ethical to conduct research that intentionally manipulates the early hormonal environment in human infants; however, there are several human disorders that act as 'experiments of nature' because they provide information about the cognitive effect of early hormone exposure. For example, several studies have examined the cognitive abilities of people living with congenital adrenal hyperplasia, an enzymatic defect that leads to high levels of androgens *in utero*. Individuals with this disorder are usually diagnosed shortly after birth and treated successfully, meaning that their postnatal hormonal environment is normal. There is preliminary evidence that females with this condition show enhanced spatial ability, which is consistent with the more masculinized cognitive profile that would be expected from their history of early androgen exposure, although not all studies are consistent in this finding. In contrast, women with Turner's syndrome have only a single X chromosome instead of the normal two, do not develop reproductive organs or female hormones, and have abnormally low levels of both androgens and estrogens. (It is normal for women to produce androgens in addition to their female hormones.) Women with Turner's syndrome have unusually poor spatial abilities, consistent with the expected effects of the low hormone levels in early life. In addition to the permanent effects of hormone exposure early in development, variations in normal adult hormone levels may have subtle effects on cognitive ability. In healthy adult men with normal androgen levels, increased amounts of testosterone in the blood are associated with better spatial ability and poorer verbal ability. In women, high estrogen levels are accompanied by relative enhancement in verbal skills, while low levels are related to relatively superior spatial abilities, even over a menstrual cycle.

Cognitive changes in response to brain injury or disease

Many studies have examined the differences between males and females in the nature and severity of cognitive deficits that develop after brain injury or neurologic disorders. These studies explore whether damage to a specific brain region causes different types of cognitive problems in men and women. The majority have looked at the cognitive effects of damage to either the left or the right hemisphere of the brain. In general, the left hemisphere is specialized for language functions and the right hemisphere is more involved in visual–spatial tasks; therefore, one would expect left hemisphere damage to result in language problems and right hemisphere damage to result in visual–spatial problems. In keeping with this expected pattern, when men with damage to the left hemisphere of the brain are given intelligence tests, they usually show a relative deficit on verbal intelligence as compared to nonverbal intelligence, whereas men with right hemisphere damage usually show the opposite pattern. In contrast, women with damage to one hemisphere do not show this well-lateralized pattern of cognitive deficits that are limited to verbal or visual functions, dependent on the hemisphere that is injured. The research findings in women, however, have not all been entirely consistent. Reports show that women generally demonstrate deficits on both verbal and nonverbal intelligence performance following left hemisphere damage, and also that women may show deficits in verbal intelligence and verbal memory following damage to either hemisphere. Men are more likely than women to develop language dysfunction (aphasia) after left hemisphere damage, although not all researchers agree.

There are several theories about why sex differences are seen after damage to one hemisphere of the brain. One theory suggests that the male brain may be more lateralized than the female brain. That is, while language may be primarily controlled by the left hemisphere in most people, this asymmetry in brain function, with the left hemisphere being more important than the right hemisphere in the control of language functions, may be more pronounced in men than in women. If language functions are represented more bilaterally (in both the left and right hemispheres) in females, women would be expected to demonstrate less severe deficits following unilateral brain lesions. Support for this theory comes from a large number of studies showing that men are more likely than women to show lateralized cognitive deficits after damage to one hemisphere of the brain. In addition, there are provocative new data using functional magnetic resonance imaging (fMRI), a noninvasive technique that measures regional blood flow changes in the brain during cognitive activity, suggesting that healthy men who perform verbal tasks are using the left hemisphere of their brains, whereas healthy women are using both the left and right hemispheres.

Sex differences in response to unilateral lesions may also result from the different strategies that men and women sometimes use when solving problems. For example, it has been reported that females generally use verbally based strategies to solve both verbal and visual–spatial or quantitative problems. If this is the case, it is not surprising to see that both verbal and non-verbal problem solving is impaired following left-sided injury in females. The preferential use of verbal strategies in women would also be consistent with their pattern of lowered performance on both verbal and nonverbal tasks after lesions in the language-dominant left hemisphere. Whether sex-related differences following brain injury are primarily due to differences in structural or functional brain organization or to differences in strategies used in the processing of cognitive abilities needs to be further investigated. For, although it is clear that males and females show structural differences in brain morphology, it is unclear how biological and environmental determinants interact to produce the sex-related differences that are seen in a number of cognitive areas.

Studies in men and women with epilepsy

Whereas most people with epilepsy have normal cognitive abilities, some have cognitive difficulties (dysfunction) related to the effects of epilepsy and seizures on the brain and the side effects of treatment. Very few studies have looked at differences in the cognitive abilities of men and women with epilepsy. People who have epilepsy because of a left hemisphere brain injury that occurs early in life (before the age of 1) may show sex differences in cognitive skills. Because the left hemisphere of the brain usually controls speech, damage to the left hemisphere often causes difficulty with language. However, a proportion of individuals who experience early left hemisphere damage go on to transfer their speech functions to the healthy right hemisphere. In the relatively few people who have language function in the right hemisphere, left hemisphere injury causes very little, if any, language problems.

The transfer of speech to the right hemisphere is typically associated with some degree of cognitive loss in areas other than language, probably because the brain regions that usually control these other functions are now forced to support language skills also. Women with epilepsy resulting from early left hemisphere lesions may have difficulties in both language and nonlanguage functions only if speech is transferred to the right hemisphere. However, men show generalized cognitive dysfunction following early left hemisphere injury regardless of whether speech is represented in the left or the right hemisphere. This suggests that women have earlier brain maturation than do men. Men have more widespread cognitive problems due to the greater immaturity of their brains at the time of injury. If injury occurs while brain cells are still developing and forming connections to other brain regions, it is more likely to cause a cascade of abnormalities, even at remote brain sites, than if there is injury to cells that have already matured and established their neural connections.

Several studies have examined whether men and women differ in their cognitive abilities after epilepsy surgery in the anterior temporal lobe. Before surgery, women are better than men at learning word lists (consistent with what is seen in healthy adults), and this sex difference persists following surgery. Men are more likely than women to show a drop in verbal memory after temporal lobe surgery (lobectomy), which is consistent with the literature suggesting that verbal skills are less lateralized in women than in men.

Less is known about sex differences in memory for visual information following temporal lobectomy. One study found that, overall, neither men nor women declined significantly following temporal lobectomy (removal of part of the temporal lobe) in their ability to remember visual material. However, those women who had a relatively larger right than left hippocampus (a temporal lobe brain structure that is critical to memory ability) before surgery had the strongest preoperative visual memory abilities and also showed the greatest memory decline following surgery. This relationship between the hippocampal size and memory loss was not apparent in men. This result may seem to be inconsistent with the data suggesting that women have less lateralized cognitive abilities than men. The authors suggest that perhaps women are more able to recover from left hemisphere lesions and men show a better ability to recover from right hemisphere lesions. This hypothesis will need to be tested in future studies that address visual memory loss following temporal lobe surgery.

Summary

Men and women have subtle but measurable differences in brain structure, cognitive ability, and brain organization. Sex differences are often not examined or reported in studies of neurologic illness and injury. Only a few studies have examined sex differences in the cognitive abilities of people with epilepsy. Preliminary evidence suggests that men and women show slightly differing cognitive symptoms in response to early brain injuries that cause epilepsy or after temporal lobe surgery to treat epilepsy. Most importantly, the existing literature suggests that more comprehensive study of the cognitive differences between men and women with epilepsy may enhance our understanding of which individuals will benefit most from specific treatment options.

SELECTED REFERENCES

Basso A, Capiani E, Moraschnini S. Sex differences in recovery from aphasia. *Cortex* 1982; 18:469–75.

Berenbaum SA, Baxter L, Seidenbberg M, Hermann B. Role of the hippocampus in sex differences in verbal memory: memory outcome following left anterior temporal lobectomy. *Neuropsychology* 1997; 11:585–91.

Christiansen K, Knussman R. Sex hormones and cognitive functioning in men. *Neuropsychobiology* 1987; 18:27–36.

Geckler C, Chelune G, Trenerry M, Ivnik R. Gender related differences in cognitive status following temporal lobectomy. *Arch Clin Neuropsychol* 1993; 138:226–7.

Gorski RA, Gordon J, Shryne JE, Southam A. Evidence for a morphological difference with the medial preoptic area of the rat brain. *Brain Res* 1978; 148:333–46.

Gur RC, Mozley LH, Mcbley PD, et al. Sex differences in regional cerebral glucose metabolism during a resting state. *Science* 1995; 267:528–31.

Halpern D. *Sex Differences in Cognitive Abilities.* Lawrence Earlbaum, Hillsdale, NJ, 1992.

Halpern DF. Sex difference in intelligence. *Am Psychol* 1997; 52:1091.

Hampson E. Variations in sex-related cognitive abilities across the menstrual cycle. *Brain Cogn* 1990; 14:26–43.

Hines M. Prenatal gonadal hormones and sex difference in human behavior. *Psychol Bull* 1982; 92:56–80.

Inglis J, Lawson JS. Sex differences in the effects of unilateral brain damage on intelligence. *Science* 1981; 212:693–5.

LeVay S. A difference in hypothalamic structure between heterosexual and homosexual men. *Science* 1991; 253:1034–7.

MacCoby EE, Jacklin CN. *The Psychology of Sex Differences.* Stanford University Press, Stanford, 1974.

McGlone J. Sex differences in human brain asymmetry: a critical survey. *Behav Brain Sci* 1980; 3:2152–3.

McGlone J. Memory complaints before and temporal lobectomy: do they predict memory performance of lesion laterality? *Epilepsia* 1994; 35:529–39.

Resnick SM, Berenbaum SA, Gottesman II, Bouchard TJ. Early hormonal influences on cognitive functioning in congenital adrenal hyperplasia. *Devel Pyschol* 1986; 22:191–8.

Shaywitz JA, Shaywitz SE, Pugh KR, et al. Sex differences in the functional organization of the brain for language. *Nature* 1995; 373:604–9.

Strauss E, Wada J, Hunter M. Sex-related differences in the cognitive consequences of early left-hemisphere lesions. *J Clin Exp Neuropsychol* 1992; 14:737–48.

Sundet K. Sex differences in cognitive impairment following unilateral brain damage. *J Clin Exp Neuropsychol* 1986; 8:51–61.

Toran-Allerand CD. Sex steroids and the development of the newborn mouse hypothalamus and preoptic area in vitro: implications for sexual differentiation. *Brain Res* 1976; 106:407–12.

Treneny MR, Clifford RTJ, Cascino GD, Sharbrough FW, Ivnik RI. Sex differences in the relationship between visual memory and MRI hippocampal volumes. *Neuropsychol* 1996; 10:343–51.

Treneny MR, Jack CRI, Cascino GD, Sharbrough FW, Ivnik RI. Gender differences in post-temporal lobectomy verbal memory and relationships between MRI hippocampal volumes and preoperative verbal memory. *Epilepsy Res* 1995; 2:69–76.

Wampson E, Kimura D. Reciprocal effects of hormonal fluctuations on human motor and perceptual–spatial skills. *Behav Neurosci* 1988; 102:456–9.

11

Sex hormones and how they act in the brain: a primer on the molecular mechanisms of action of sex steroid hormones

Philip A. Schwartzkroin

Women with epilepsy have known for some time that female hormones affect seizures. Scientists have only recently begun to understand why this is so. Hormones impact brain function in many ways. Female sex hormones change the excitability of brain neurons by increasing excitation or inhibition. These hormones act on the cell membrane, changing the threshold for firing, change the rate at which neurons manufacture excitatory and inhibitory brain chemicals, and even change the shape of neurons, altering the way brain cells connect to one another.

Dr Philip Schwartzkroin addresses this fascinating and complex topic. Dr Schwartzkroin is a PhD in Neuroscience and is a Professor of Neuroscience at the University of California Davis, where he heads a laboratory that studies how epilepsy develops in the brain. Further research into the science of hormone effects on brain neurons will lead to better understanding of epilepsy and, most certainly, to new treatments.

MJM

Scientists have long known that steroid sex hormones – those hormones that are made in the ovaries in women and in the testes in men – are critical elements in reproductive and other sexual behaviors. We are only beginning to understand, however, that these same hormones can exert influences on regions of the brain that have little to do – at least directly – with sexual/reproductive activity. These effects on the brain have been best studied for the female hormones – progesterone and estrogen – partly as a result of the fact that in some women with epilepsy, seizure occurrence appears to be related to parts of the menstrual cycle when estrogen levels are highest and progesterone levels are lowest.

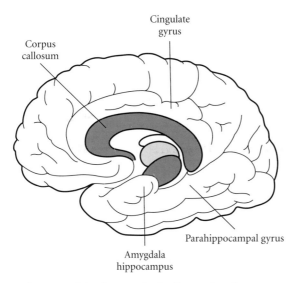

Figure 11.1 A diagram of the human brain illustrating the corpus callosum, the major pathway connecting the left and right activity between several brain regions, and the amygdala and hippocampus, areas involved in temporal lobe epilepsy.

We certainly are aware that in human beings mental processes can affect sexual and reproductive activities. Given that information, we might well guess that those parts of our brain that are particularly involved in mental processing – the cerebral cortex and the hippocampus (a brain structure often associated with learning and memory functions) – can exert a significant influence over the brain circuits involved in sexual functions (Fig. 11.1).

These latter circuits – which involve the hypothalamus, the pituitary, and the gonads – are arranged in a 'feedback' circuit (Fig. 11.2). The cerebral cortex and hippocampus detect the levels of circulating sex hormones and modulate the circuit to produce more or less hormone output.

The sensors employed by cells in the brain are called 'receptors.' Receptors are complex molecules that 'recognize' a hormone or neurotransmitter. When the hormone combines with its receptor, it initiates a complex series of 'signalling' events that result in changes in activity and/or metabolism of the nerve cell. The receptor can thus 'transduce' the presence of significant levels of hormone into a physiologically meaningful signal. There appear to be at least two distinct types of hormone receptors in the brain.

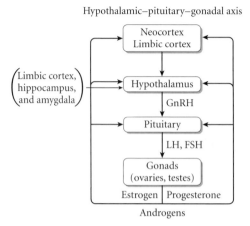

Figure 11.2 A block diagram showing the major components of the circuit involved in brain modulation of hormone secretion from the gonads – and of the feedback via gonadal hormones to the central nervous system. Although it has long been clear that the hypothalamus and pituitary are critically involved in reproductive behavior, we are just beginning to understand how gonadal hormones, such as estrogen and progesterone, affect the functioning of neurons in 'higher' brain regions. (GnRH = gonadotropin-releasing hormone; LH = luteinizing hormone; FSH = follicle-stimulating hormone.)

The first type is the receptor type generally associated with steroid hormones, and specifically with the reproductive and sexual function of female steroid sex hormones. Steroid molecules such as estrogen and progesterone easily pass through the cell membrane and are able to find receptor molecules within the cell (Fig. 11.3). The hormone–receptor complex then binds to a specific site on the DNA in the cell's nucleus, and controls the genetic activity of the cell (transcription). For example, progesterone acts on hypothalamic cells to alter the gene responsible for the production of gonadotropin-releasing hormone (GnRH) – the substance responsible for triggering the release of luteinizing hormone (LH) and follicle-stimulating hormone (FH) from the pituitary. These gene changes take a long time, and the delay from hormone–receptor binding to synthesis of the gene product (protein) may take hours or days.

However, we now know that sex hormones can exert much faster effects – effects that occur so quickly that they could not possibly involve gene transcription and protein synthesis. Such effects are mediated, we think, by

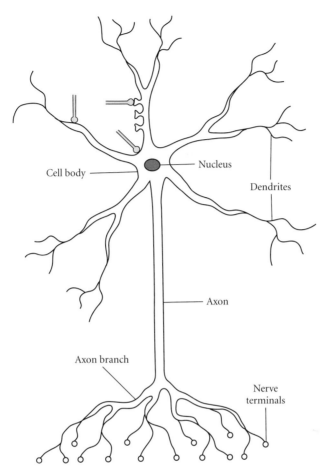

Figure 11.3 The structure of a typical neuron. The dendrites contain synapses that communicate from cell to cell.

receptors that sit within the cell membrane (Fig. 11.3). Such receptors may control channels for electrically charged molecules and/or modulate the function of other receptors – all without involving the genetic machinery. It is thought that some of the actions of progesterone and estrogen that affect the *excitability* of nerve cells – and thus may influence epileptic seizures – are controlled via such membrane-bound receptors.

What is the evidence that these ovarian steroid hormonal actions do, in fact, alter the excitability of the brain and alter the threshold for seizures? There are dozens of suggestive studies in animals with epilepsy that support this point of view. For example, estrogen treatment appears to increase the number of receptors available to bind excitatory neurotransmitters. Further, investigators have shown that electrically stimulated neuronal excitation is enhanced by estrogen but dampened by progesterone. Also, learning and memory, which require activity of brain neurons, appear to be facilitated by estrogen treatment. Studies of the factors that cause epilepsy also show that female steroid hormones affect brain excitability. Over 35 years ago, a group of researchers found that estradiol (the primary form of estrogen produced by human ovaries) administered to rats lowered the threshold for epileptic seizures. Rats treated with estradiol exhibited seizures at lower levels of seizure-inducing drugs (or of other treatments) than rats not treated with estrogen. Other experiments have shown that estradiol itself can induce seizure-like electrical activities. In contrast, progesterone breakdown products not only decrease seizure severity in animals, but also appear to protect the brain from damage that often results from repetitive seizures.

These studies indicate that either progesterone or estrogen, or both, may influence the occurrence of epileptic seizures. Of major interest is how estrogen and progesterone exert these effects.

Progesterone – and especially some of its metabolites – can depress brain excitability, and therefore may reduce seizure activity. When progesterone is metabolized in the body, a specific set of breakdown products – now often called 'neuroactive steroids' – can have powerful effects on nerve cells. Further, it appears that similar molecules – 'neurosteroids' – can actually be manufactured in the brain, in the 'support' cells or glia. These steroid molecules bind to a receptor that is involved in the majority of inhibitory interactions among neurons – the GABA receptor. This receptor is the 'sensor' for gamma aminobutyric acid (GABA), the principal inhibitory neurotransmitter in the brain. When GABA binds to its receptor, a set of electrical changes occurs in the cell that decreases the likelihood that the cell will be active (i.e., discharge an electrical impulse, or 'action potential'). One way to quiet the brain, to decrease its activity, is to enhance the effectiveness of GABA at its receptor – to increase inhibition. Many of the currently used antiepileptic drugs work in this way, for example diazepam (Valium). Now researchers have found that some neuroactive metabolites of progesterone affect the GABA receptor in a way quite similar to the antiepileptic drugs diazepam, lorazepam, clonazepam, phenobarbital, and primidone. This action of neuroactive steroids is rapid (fractions of seconds), and easily reversible. As might be expected from this similarity to the diazepam family of medications, the progesterone metabolites have a number of additional effects, including anti-anxiety effects and sedation. Given such actions, investigators are trying to develop new antiepileptic drugs based on these progesterone-derived steroids that will be antiepileptic but without the other significant side effects.

The other major female sex steroid hormone – estrogen – has an almost opposite effect from progesterone. Estrogen has been found to increase brain excitability. The most direct, fastest, and most obvious effect of estrogen is to increase the excitatory neurotransmitters in brain regions such as the hippocampus which are thought to be responsible for the generation of temporal lobe seizures. Estrogen is also known to alter the inhibitory neurotransmitter dopamine. Although it is not immediately obvious how this action affects net brain excitability, it does seem quite likely that such an effect may be quite important in the spread and generalization of seizure activity throughout the brain.

One final example of the potential important effects of estrogen and progesterone on brain function – and structure – is worth mentioning. Recently, researchers found that estrogen may actually alter the structural elements of neurons that are involved in cell-to-cell communication – the synapses, (Fig. 11.4). A synapse is composed of two primary elements: (1) the presynaptic terminal, which contains a neurotransmitter that is released from

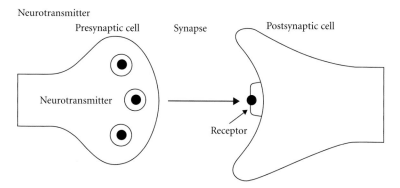

Figure 11.4 Neurotransmiters are released from presynaptic cells into the synapse to stimulate receptors on postsynaptic cells at very close range.

the cell when that neuron discharges; and (2) the postsynaptic *spine*, which contains the receptor molecules that respond to transmitters released from the presynaptic cell.

Investigators studying female rats have found that during the part of the estrous cycle when estrogen is high (proestrus), there is an increase – of 20–30% – in the number of synaptic contacts between presynaptic and post-synaptic elements. Such a dramatic change in nerve cell structure has an effect on neuron-to-neuron communication. These changes – relatively rapid, dramatic, and reversible – may help to explain some of the pro-seizure effects seen in women during certain parts of their menstrual cycle.

Whereas we believe that progesterone is an inhibitory agent and estrogen is an excitatory agent, it is important to be aware that these two hormones may – and often do – act together. Indeed, they normally rise and fall in a highly coordinated manner that makes it important to understand their interactions. Experimental studies suggest that their actions together are not simple sums of their separate effects. To better understand their actions, and to treat the seizure-related effects of steroid hormone fluctuation, we must gain a better understanding of how, and where, these hormones interact.

SELECTED REFERENCES

Majewska MD. Neurosteroids: endogenous bimodal modulators of the GABA-A receptor. Mechanism of action and physiological significance. *Progr Neurobiol* 1992; 38:379–95.

McEwen BS, Coirini H, Westlind-Danielsson A, et al. Steroid hormones as mediators of neural plasticity. *J Steroid Biochem Mol Biol* 1991; 39:223–32.

Morrell MJ Hormones and epilepsy through the lifetime. *Epilepsia* 1992; 33 (Suppl. 4):S49–S61.

Terasawa E, Timiras PS. Electrical activity during the estrous cycle of the rat: cyclic changes in limbic structures. *Endocrinology* 1968; 83:207–16.

12

Epilepsy and the menstrual cycle

Patricia O. Shafer and Andrew G. Herzog

Many women with epilepsy find that seizures are more likely to occur at certain times of the menstrual cycle. Menstrual-associated seizure patterns (called catamenial seizures) have been written about in medical textbooks for hundreds of years. We finally understand why these seizure patterns exist. As Dr Herzog and Ms Shafer discuss, fluctuations in the levels of the hormones estrogen and progesterone over the menstrual cycle cause changes in brain excitability. This changes the seizure threshold. Generally, seizures are most likely to occur in the days preceding the onset of menstrual flow and at the time of ovulation. Understanding seizure and hormone relationships could lead to new treatments. Some trials of hormone therapies in women with menstrual-associated seizures are now underway.

Dr Andrew Herzog is an Associate Professor of Neurology at Harvard Medical School. He has received funding from the National Institutes of Health for his research into hormone effects on seizures. He was truly one of the pioneers in this field and continues to be an active researcher, author, and lecturer. Dr Herzog serves on the Epilepsy Foundation Professional Advisory Board. Ms Patricia Osborne Shafer is an Epilepsy Clinical Nurse Specialist at Beth Israel Deaconess Medical Center. She has been active in the Epilepsy Foundation in a number of capacities, most recently as a member of the National Board of Directors and as incoming Head of the Professional Advisory Board. In this chapter, these two highly qualified individuals provide information about this important topic.

MJM

Do seizures occur more frequently around the time of menstruation? Is there a physical cause, or is it 'all in my head?' These are just a few of the questions that many women have been asking for centuries. Published reports of menstrual cycle irregularities in association with seizures date to 1870. A 1996 survey of women contacting the Epilepsy Foundation affiliates reveals that 53% of respondents reported having problems, ranging from 'some' to 'significant' problems, with changes in their seizures in relation to their menses, while 49% reported irregular menses as a concern. Unfortunately, 46% of respondents felt that their doctor did not take their concerns seriously.

Fortunately, there have been many advances in our understanding of seizures and hormones in recent years. We now know that, in some women, hormonal changes can alter the frequency or pattern of seizures, and that there is a greater incidence of menstrual cycle problems in some women with epilepsy. The purpose of this chapter is to provide an overview of the normal menstrual cycle and what changes may be seen in women with epilepsy. Catamenial epilepsy is explained, as well as the effects of seizures and medications on menstruation and of hormonal changes on seizures.

What happens in normal menstruation?

About every 28 days, a woman's body undergoes complex hormonal changes, which result in menstruation. The menstrual bleeding occurs from sloughing of the lining of the uterus. The menstrual cycle is under the control of the hypothalamus, a specialized region of the brain, which secretes luteinizing hormone-releasing hormone (LHRH), by which it regulates the secretion of hormones by the pituitary gland. A pituitary hormone called the follicle-stimulating hormone (FSH) acts on the ovary during the first half of the menstrual cycle to induce egg development and release (ovulation) by mid-cycle. Another pituitary hormone called luteinizing hormone (LH) acts on the ovary to produce and secrete estrogen and, in the second half of the cycle after ovulation, progesterone as well as estrogen. A critical level of estrogen is necessary during the first half of the cycle for ovulation to occur. If the released egg comes in contact with sperm, the fertilized egg makes its way to the uterus and settles in the lining (the endometrium). Estrogen and progesterone are needed in the second half of the cycle to thicken the endometrium for implantation. If all this occurs successfully, a woman will become pregnant and the fertilized egg will develop into a fetus and then a baby. If the egg is not fertilized or does not get implanted into the lining of the uterus, the body sheds the thickened uterine lining by the process known as menstrual bleeding.

As one can see, hormones are instrumental in the monthly process of menstruation. The ovarian hormones (estrogen, progesterone, and some testosterone) need to be present in a woman's body for menstruation to

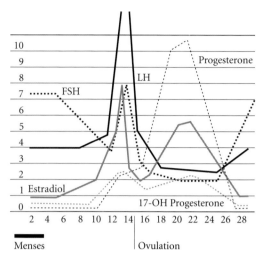

Figure 12.1 The normal menstrual cycle.

proceed normally. The amount of each hormone varies at different times of the menstrual cycle. For example, in the middle of the cycle, the level of estrogen is highest, and triggers ovulation. After ovulation, a surge of progesterone occurs, which relates to the preparation of the uterus for the egg. Shortly before menstruation, the levels of both estrogen and progesterone drop, stimulating the process of menstrual bleeding. Figure 12.1 demonstrates the typical variations in estradiol (a form of estrogen) and progesterone levels during menstruation.

A menstrual cycle typically lasts 28 days, but there is wide variation among women. Day 1 of the cycle is the first day of menstrual bleeding, and ovulation typically occurs 14 days before the onset of the next menstruation. In the middle of a 28-day cycle, this would be around day 14. The premenstrual period is usually considered to be a few days before menstruation, but may range to a week or 10 days preceding menstruation, or days 18 to 28. When menstruation begins again, the counting of the menstrual cycle begins again at day 1.

What changes in menstrual cycles occur in women with epilepsy?

One-third to one-half of women with temporal lobe epilepsy report menstrual cycle problems. These include going several months without menstruation (amenorrhea), having menstrual cycles longer than 35 days (oligomenorrhea), or unusually long (greater than 32 days) or short (less than 26 days) times between menstrual periods. Ovulation does not occur (anovulatory cycles) and, therefore, progesterone is not secreted during the second half of the cycle (inadequate luteal phase cycles) in approximately 35% of cycles in women with temporal lobe epilepsy, as compared to about 7% among women in the general population (Cummings et al., 1995). Women with the above-listed menstrual disorders are more likely to have anovulatory and inadequate luteal phase cycles. These cycles usually result from abnormal hormone secretion and are associated with increased seizure frequency.

Some of these menstrual cycle problems are the result of distinct reproductive endocrine disorders, which involve the production of abnormal quantities of reproductive hormones. Polycystic ovarian syndrome (PCOS) and hypothalamic amenorrhea are examples of reproductive endocrine disorders that are thought to occur more frequently in women with partial epilepsy. Exactly how frequently these problems occur is not yet known; however, Herzog et al. suggest that PCOS (which involves the occurrence of menstrual disorders, excess hair growth, and small cysts in the ovaries associated with elevated serum levels of androgens – masculinizing hormones) occurs in about 20% of women with temporal lobe epilepsy, as compared to 5% of the general population. Hypothalamic amenorrhea (characterized by menstrual disorders, including loss of menses, associated with low pituitary FSH and LH as well as low estrogen levels) occurs in about 12% of women with temporal lobe epilepsy, as compared to 1.5% of the general population. Both of these epilepsy-related conditions are associated with inadequate luteal phase cycles, which can result in infertility and increased seizure occurrence.

Some researchers believe that certain seizure medications may contribute to menstrual cycle problems. It is not unusual for women who change medications to experience a change in their menstrual periods. This type of change is often temporary, and once their body gets used to the new medicine, the menstrual periods become more regular. Other women notice changes that persist for a period of time and can be bothersome. We know that some medications taken for mood or thought disorders, such as depression, may affect menstrual cycles. Sodium valproate, used for both seizures and mood disorders, has been associated with long periods of time without menstruation and possibly with a greater chance of developing PCOS.

It is not definitely known whether the medication makes a woman more likely to have this condition, or if the underlying seizure disorder is the cause. Other medications have not been studied exclusively for their effect on menstruation in women with epilepsy.

What is catamenial epilepsy?

Catamenial epilepsy is a term that has been used for many years to describe the pattern of seizures occurring around menstruation. Typically, catamenial seizures were thought to occur only immediately before or during menstruation. Herzog et al. now propose three patterns of catamenial seizures. Information was collected from 184 women with uncontrolled seizures by charting seizures and menstrual cycles and measuring day 22 progesterone levels. A seizure exacerbation in this study was defined as seizures occurring at least twice as often as usual. Two different patterns were seen most often in women with normal menstrual cycles: seizures occurring before or during the first few days of menstruation and seizures at the time of ovulation. A third pattern of seizure exacerbation, which occurred during the entire second half of the menstrual cycle, was seen in women who had abnormal menstrual cycles and did not ovulate regularly. Figure 12.2 shows these patterns of catamenial epilepsy in relation to levels of estradiol and progesterone.

What are the causes of catamenial seizures?

Both estrogen and progesterone affect the excitability of brain cells, especially in the temporal and frontal lobes of the brain. Estrogen can make seizures more likely to occur, whereas progesterone can decrease or inhibit seizure activity. Normally, estrogen levels are higher than progesterone levels in the days leading up to ovulation and immediately before menstrual bleeding. These are the times in the menstrual cycle during which many women notice more frequent and/or more severe seizures (especially just before menstruation). If a woman has menstrual cycles in which she does not ovulate, she may not have enough progesterone during the entire second half of the menstrual cycle. During anovulatory cycles, seizures may be worse for the entire second half of the cycle.

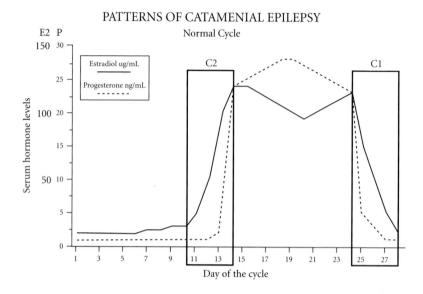

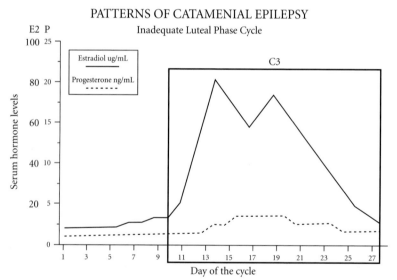

Figure 12.2 Three patterns of catamenial epilepsy. (From Herzog AG, Klein P, Ransil BJ. Three patterns of catamenial epilepsy. *Epilepsia* 1997; 38 (10):1083.

Hormones from the hypothalamus and pituitary gland regulate the amount of estrogen and progesterone circulating in a woman's body. The hypothalamus, in turn, receives many direct connections from those parts of the temporal lobe that are involved in the generation of seizures. Research has shown that seizure discharges in these areas can disrupt the output of hormones such as FSH and LH, which in turn can alter the balance of estrogen and progesterone and affect seizure control. In other words, seizures can affect hormones, and hormone levels can also affect seizures.

Varying levels of seizure medications may also contribute to catamenial seizures. Estrogen and progesterone are metabolized (broken down) by the same liver enzymes that metabolize most of the commonly used seizure medications (phenytoin, carbamazepine, phenobarbital, primidone, and topiramate). Estrogen and progesterone levels change throughout the menstrual cycle. Hormonal concentrations at different times of the menstrual cycle can affect the speed and manner in which the liver breaks down these seizure medicines. For example, premenstrually – when the levels of estrogen and progesterone are low – more of the liver enzymes are free to metabolize these antiepileptic medications, resulting in lower levels of antiepileptic medication in the body than normal. If this situation occurs, the woman would be more likely to have seizures at that time.

How can I tell if seizures are affected by menstrual cycles?

The easiest way to determine if seizures are related to the menstrual cycle is to record the occurrence and type of seizures and the day menstruation starts on a calendar. The more information one can record, the easier it will be to see changes or patterns. For example, if a woman is able to tell when she ovulates, changes in seizures can be noticed at that time as well. Some women can tell they are ovulating because of the presence of mid-cycle vaginal discharges or changes in their basal body temperature in the middle of the cycle. Recording a basal body temperature is done by checking one's temperature first thing in the morning before eating and before getting out of bed. A blood test can also be done on day 22 of the menstrual period to measure the amount of progesterone in the body. Other details concerning the menstrual cycle can be helpful, for example if there are changes in the length or type of menstrual bleeding, cramping or other discomfort. Counting the first day of menstruation as day 1 then counting forward until the menstrual bleeding begins again determines the length of the menstrual cycle. It is helpful to record the day of the menstrual cycle on

INSTRUCTIONS: Please place the date in the upper left hand corner for each day. Complete each day with the number of seizures you had. Refer to the **SEIZURE CODES** to make recording easier and shorter. Please write any changes in seizures or medications, use of non-seizure medications, or possible triggers of seizures such as missed or extra medication doses, alcohol or other drug use, fatigue, lack of sleep, illness, emotional stress, and/or external stimuli (i.e., loud noises, music, lights, etc.).

FEMALES ONLY: Please record the day of your menstrual cycle in the top right hand corner of each box. The first day of your period should be counted as day 1 of your cycle. Record changes in menstruation, dates of hormonal treatment (e.g., progesterone), and any changes in mood, seizures, or behavior.

SAMPLE

FOUR-WEEK SEIZURE CALENDAR

Name: **Beth Israel Hospital**
Beth Israel#:   **Comprehensive Epilepsy Center**

Sunday	Monday	Tuesday	Wednesday	Thursday	Friday	Saturday
Date: 1 Cycle: 26	Date: 2 Cycle: 27 1 - I Have flu. Temp. = 101°F Took 2 Tylenol.	Date: 3 Cycle: 1 3 - I's Period started.	Date: 4 Cycle: 2 3 - I's Flu little better today Total Seizures: 3	Date: 5 Cycle: 3	Date: 6 Cycle: 4	Date: 7 Cycle: 5 2 - I's 1 - II Forgot a. m. meds
Total Seizures: 0	Total Seizures: 1	Total Seizures: 3		Total Seizures: 2	Total Seizures: O	Total Seizures: 3
Date:____ Cycle:____	Date:____ Cycle:____	Date:____ Cycle:____	Date:____ Cycle:____	Date:____ Cycle:____	Date:____ Cycle:____	Date:____ Cycle:____
Total Seizures:	Total Seizures:	Total Seizures:	Total Seizures:	Total Seizures:	Total Seizures:	Total Seizures:
Date:____ Cycle:____	Date:____ Cycle:____	Date:____ Cycle:____	Date:____ Cycle:____	Date:____ Cycle:____	Date:____ Cycle:____	Date:____ Cycle:____
Total Seizures:	Total Seizures:	Total Seizures:	Total Seizures:	Total Seizures:	Total Seizures:	Total Seizures:
Date:____ Cycle:____	Date:____ Cycle:____	Date:____ Cycle:____	Date:____ Cycle:____	Date:____ Cycle:____	Date:____ Cycle:____	Date:____ Cycle:____
Total Seizures:	Total Seizures:	Total Seizures:	Total Seizures:	Total Seizures:	Total Seizures:	Total Seizures:

MEDICATIONS: **SEIZURE CODES:**

Dilantin (200/200 mg)   I = Funny feeling in head

Tegretol (200/200/300 mg)   II = Funny feeling in head, then blackout.

TOTAL NUMBER OF SEIZURES FOR THIS MONTH:_____   AVERAGE NUMBER OF SEIZURES PER DAY:_____

Figure 12.3 Monthly seizure calendar. (From the Comprehensive Epilepsy Center, Beth Israel Deaconess Medical Center, Boston, MA.)

the same calendar as the seizures. An example of a seizure calendar is shown in Figure 12.3.

Information about other factors that can affect a woman's seizures and menses should be noted. For example, missed medication, sleep deprivation, stress, intense or excessive exercise, poor appetite or intake, or excessive caffeine may influence seizures or menses in some women. Whereas some people with seizures are aware of predictable triggers to their seizures, others notice no changes or only changes in their seizures when more than one factor occurs at the same time. Examining this information over time can help the woman and her doctor or nurse detect whether there is a predictable pattern to her seizures.

Once she has recorded information from at least three menstrual cycles, a woman should review this with her doctor or nurse. If a pattern is present, the doctor may recommend further testing to see if a hormonal imbalance is present or if medication levels change during certain times of the menstrual cycle. Blood tests of certain hormones can be done at two times during the menstrual cycle, around day 4 and again around day 22. A gynecological evaluation is helpful to see if there are any conditions such as ovarian cysts, fertility problems, or menopause that could be contributing to menstrual cycle problems and seizures. Tests such as a pelvic ultrasound may be ordered specifically to look at the ovaries and uterus.

To find out whether medications are part of the problem, blood tests can be done to detect the level of antiepileptic medications. These tests need to be done at the same time of the day (preferably before the first morning dose of medication) during menstrual bleeding and at another phase of the cycle for comparison to see if the seizure medicine concentration drops during menstruation to account for seizure exacerbation at that time. If a drop is detected, adjusting the dose of medicine at that time can be helpful.

If hormonal problems are suspected or found, a referral to an endocrinologist or a neuroendocrinologist (a specialist in hormone and neurological disorders such as epilepsy) may be helpful. These doctors can work with the neurologist to sort out the problem and see whether correcting the hormone disorder may help seizure control.

What treatments are available for catamenial epilepsy?

Progesterone therapy may be helpful for some women with catamenial seizures. There are several ways that progesterone can be given. Supplemental natural progesterone may be provided during the second half of each cycle. In one study of eight women who had inadequate luteal phase cycles with catamenial seizure exacerbation, six experienced improved seizure control with natural progesterone. In a subsequent investigation of cyclic natural progesterone, 19 of 25 women (76%) experienced fewer seizures, with an overall average monthly decline of 54% for complex partial and 58% for secondary generalized seizures over 3 months.

Natural progesterone is available as a plant extract in lozenge and capsule forms in 100–200 mg dosages and should be administered three times daily because its time of action is generally in the range of about 6 hours. The daily regimen to achieve effective blood levels generally ranges from 100 to 200 mg, taken three times daily. The usual optimal daily dose ranges from 300–600 mg. The dosage amount and time should be individualized – based on a combination of seizure response and serum progesterone levels between 5 and 25 ng/mL. Progesterone is usually administered in full dose three times daily on days 14 through 25 of each cycle. It is then reduced to half the dose on days 26 and 27, a quarter of the dose on day 28, and then discontinued. Sometimes it may be administered only during the period of seizure exacerbation, toward the end of the second half of the cycle, although this tends to be less effective.

Adverse effects occur with higher dosage and include sedation, mental depression, and tiredness. Progesterone use may also occasionally be associated with breast tenderness, weight gain, and irregular vaginal bleeding. The vehicle used to dissolve progesterone for suppository use may, rarely, cause an allergic rash. Discontinuation of the hormone or lowering of the dosage resolves these side effects.

Synthetic progestin therapy has also benefited some women with epilepsy. Intramuscular depomedroxyprogesterone significantly lessens seizure frequency when it is given in sufficient dosage to induce amenorrhea. A regimen of approximately 120–150 mg given intramuscularly every 6–12 weeks generally achieves this goal. Side effects include those encountered with natural progesterone. Depot administration, however, is also commonly associated with irregular breakthrough vaginal bleeding and a lengthy delay of 6–12 months in the return of regular ovulatory cycles. Oral synthetic progestins administered cyclically or continuously have not proven to be an effective therapy in clinical investigations, although individual successes with continuous daily oral use of norethistrone and combination pills have been reported.

There are no definite absolute clinical contraindications to the intermittent use of natural progesterone to achieve physiological luteal range serum levels in a cyclic fashion. It is used in women without epilepsy as a treatment for an inadequate luteal phase and is regularly used to help induce fertility. However, neither intermittent nor continuous progesterone therapy is recognized as an approved form of therapy for neurological purposes. Therefore, more typical antiepileptic medications should be tried first. Progesterone should be avoided (1) during or in anticipation of pregnancy, unless it is specifically used with the approval of a gynecologist as part of a fertility program, and (2) in the absence of adequate birth control measures. It should also be used cautiously in the presence of undiagnosed breast lumps because synthetic progestin use has been associated with breast nodule development and, in high doses, malignancy in experimental animals.

Drug interactions are an important consideration. Higher progesterone dosages may be required to achieve luteal range levels in women who take some antiepileptic medications that enhance the liver enzymes that metabolize steroid hormones and increase their binding (attachment) to proteins in the bloodstream (phenytoin, carbamazepine, phenobarbital, topiramate). Progesterone use has not typically been associated with changes in antiepileptic medication levels. However, antiepileptic medication levels should be checked periodically while taking and while not taking progesterone.

It is likely that progesterone has more than one effect on the brain that serves to inhibit seizures. Several mechanisms have been proposed (Herzog, 1995):

- Progesterone exerts a depressant effect on oxygen and glucose metabolism.
- Progesterone acts directly on the cortex (brain cells) to suppress seizure discharges.
- Progesterone acts indirectly via metabolites that have potent depressant effects.
- Progesterone acts indirectly to enhance brain inhibition by the brain chemical GABA.
- Progesterone acts indirectly through competition with antiepileptic medications for sites of hepatic inactivation.
- Progesterone acts indirectly by potentiating the effects of antiepileptic brain chemicals such as adenosine.
- Combinations of mechanisms are, of course, not ruled out and appear likely.

Summary

Health-care professionals who treat women with epilepsy now better understand the relationship between seizures and hormones. Research is beginning into hormonal therapies for epilepsy. Understanding each woman's seizure patterns and any hormonal association requires close collaboration between the woman with seizures and her health-care providers. Obtaining as much information as possible about seizures and menses can assist the woman and her health-care team in this process.

SELECTED REFERENCES

Cummings LN, Giudice L, Morrell MJ. Ovulatory function in epilepsy. *Epilepsia* 1995; 35: 353–7.

Drislane FW, Coleman AE, Schomer DL, et al. Altered pulsatile secretion of luteinizing hormone in women with epilepsy. *Neurology* 1994; 44:306–10.

Gonzalez Echeverria M. *On Epilepsy: Anatamo-Pathological and Clinical Notes*. William Wood & Co, New York; 1870, pp. 293–6.

Herzog AG. Intermittent progesterone therapy and frequency of complex partial seizures in women with menstrual disorders. *Neurology* 1986; 45:1607–10.

Herzog AG. Progesterone in seizure therapy. *Neurology* 1987; 37:1433.

Herzog AG. Progesterone therapy in women with complex partial and secondary generalized seizures. *Neurology* 1995; 45:1660–2.

Herzog AG, Klein P, Ransil BJ. Three patterns of catamenial epilepsy. *Epilepsia* 1997; 38(10):1082–8.

Herzog AG, Seibel MM, Schomer DL, et al. Reproductive endocrine disorders in women with partial seizures of temporal lobe origin. *Arch Neurol* 1986; 43:341–6.

Isojarvi JIT, Laatikainen TJ, Pakarinen AJ, et al. Polycystic ovaries and hyperandrogenism in women taking valproate for epilepsy. *N Engl J Med* 1993; 329:1383–8.

Klein P, Herzog AG. Endocrine aspects of partial epilepsy. In *The Comprehensive Evaluation and Treatment of Epilepsy – A Practical Guide*, ed. SC Schachter, DL Schomer. Academic Press, Boston; 1997, pp. 207–32.

Mattson RH, Cramer JA, Caldwell BV, Siconolfi BC. Treatment of seizures with medroxyprogesterone acetate: preliminary report. *Neurology* 1984; 34:1255–8.

Women and Epilepsy Initiative – Affiliate Survey. *Epilepsy USA* 1996; xxix(2). Epilepsy Foundation of America.

13

Menopause and epilepsy

Fariha Abbasi and Allan Krumholz

A woman today is likely to spend half her life after menopause. Because many types of epilepsy are life-long, this means that many women with epilepsy can expect their epilepsy treatment to continue through the menopausal years. It is surprising, therefore, that there is so little information about how menopause affects seizure control. Of particular concern is whether hormone replacement therapy might affect seizures.

Fortunately, all this is about to change. A small group of dedicated physicians is conducting research into epilepsy after menopause. One group of these researchers has provided this chapter. Dr Krumholz is Professor of Neurology at the University of Maryland and Director of the Epilepsy Center there. He is very involved in the Epilepsy Foundation, both as a former member of the National Board of Directors and on the board of his local Epilepsy Foundation affiliate. Dr Abbasi is also an epilepsy specialist trained at the University of Maryland and is now working at the Neurological Center in Gastonia, North Carolina. Although we cannot provide all the answers to questions about epilepsy after menopause, at least we are finally asking the questions.

MJM

Introduction

Menopause (the phase of a woman's life when the ovaries cease to function and menstruation stops) marks the end of a woman's natural ability to bear children. Generally occurring between the ages of 48 and 55 years, menopause is recognized as an increasingly vital and critical part of a modern woman's life. The average American woman can today expect to live approximately 30 years after menopause – about one-third of her life – and should remain active and productive through most of this period. Menopausal women are part of the fastest growing component of our society. The population of women over the age of 60 is expected to double within the next decade and issues affecting this population, such as menopause, will be of increasing importance in future years.

For women with epilepsy, menopause is an especially significant concern. Characteristically, epilepsy begins at a young age, and it is often a lifelong issue. Because epilepsy does not usually shorten the life span, a woman with epilepsy will spend about one-third of her life after menopause. Whereas the relationships between epilepsy and some phases of a woman's reproductive life, such as pregnancy, are known to be of considerable importance, much less is known about the associations of epilepsy with menopause. Therefore, it is extremely important that women with epilepsy and their physicians be aware of the potential effects of menopause on epilepsy to ensure the best quality of life in the later years. This chapter reviews the issues women face regarding menopause and discuss what is known about the influence of menopause on epilepsy and seizures.

Natural history of menopause

Hormones such as estrogen and progesterone influence the brain at birth and help establish sexual differentiation between men and women. Estrogen is the most important hormone in female development; testosterone has a central role in male development. Throughout childhood, these hormones prepare the body for sexual maturity: in women, this maturity is marked by the beginning of the menstrual cycle, typically 2 years after the onset of puberty. The menstrual cycle varies from 25 to 30 days, during which time the ovaries are stimulated, estrogen is produced, and ovulation (egg production) occurs. If the egg is not fertilized and pregnancy does not occur, the egg released in ovulation dies and hormonal levels of estrogen and another important female hormone, progesterone, fall. The uterus, which had been prepared by these hormones to accept a fertilized egg, responds to this fall in hormones by shedding its lining with the menstrual flow. The same 25–30-day cycle begins all over again.

As a woman ages, this process continues until the eggs and hormone-producing cells in the ovary are exhausted. When the ovaries cease to produce viable eggs and estrogen secretion declines, the cycle is interrupted and menstruation stops. In most women, these changes are gradual, often accompanied by troubling symptoms such as hot flashes (or flushes), night sweats, mood swings, headaches, and dry skin. This transitional stage, known as the perimenopausal phase, may last for several years until menstruation stops completely. Women whose menopause results from a surgical hysterectomy with removal of the ovaries are also menopausal and may have many of the same problems.

Women naturally undergo menopause at the average age of about 51 years; this process is unaffected by factors such as race and socioeconomic status. Only cigarette smoking has been shown to accelerate the loss of ovarian follicles and the onset of menopause.

Body changes associated with menopause

Although menopause is a natural part of the aging process, it can still cause problems for women. The low estrogen levels that are a part of menopause affect many different organ systems in the body. These changes generally occur slowly and differ for each woman: whereas some women hardly notice any difficulties, others find the problems of menopause severe and debilitating. Table 13.1 lists some of the reported adverse effects of menopause, which are discussed below.

Vascular autonomic changes

Hot flashes are experienced by 75–85% of all menopausal women. These sudden feelings of intense heat spread over the body and may be associated with severe perspiration or sweating. The hot flash can vary in severity among individuals from a minor symptom to an incapacitating problem. These symptoms occur most commonly at night, in warm environments, after ingestion of alcohol or spicy foods, and during periods of stress. The hot flashes last from a few minutes up to several hours; episodes usually repeat for several months and then improve. In some cases, however, hot flashes persist for years. Fortunately, particularly troubling hot flashes can be treated successfully with hormone replacement therapy (HRT) with estrogen.

Heart disease

Estrogen lowers the risk of heart disease throughout a woman's reproductive years. After menopause, and with decreasing estrogen levels, this risk increases substantially. Because heart disease occurs at a younger age in men,

Table 13.1. Problems associated
with menopause

Vascular autonomic changes
    Hot flashes (flushes)
    Severe sweating
Cardiovascular disease
    Heart attacks
    Strokes
Bone disorders
    Osteoporosis
    Broken bones
    Hip fractures
Vaginal and urinary tract problems
    Vaginal irritation
    Urinary infections
Sleep difficulties
Emotional symptoms

it has been thought of as mainly a male problem, and its prevention and treatment in women have been somewhat neglected. Heart disease is, however, still the most common cause of death in women and kills twice as many women as cancer. Fortunately, good strategies are developing to prevent and treat heart disease in women.

For example, there is good evidence that HRT can reduce the risk of heart attacks in menopausal women, particularly those with major risks for heart disease. Factors that contribute to this risk include a family history of heart disease, abnormalities in cholesterol and lipids, high blood pressure, diabetes, and cigarette smoking. When a woman considers the use of HRT in menopause, she and her physician should carefully assess her risk for heart disease (Fig. 13.1).

Bone disorders and osteoporosis

Excessive bone loss can cause a thinning of the bone called osteoporosis. This disorder puts a woman at major risk for broken bones and serious fractures, such as hip fractures, which are associated with a high death rate. Osteoporosis is a particular problem for menopausal women, who are well

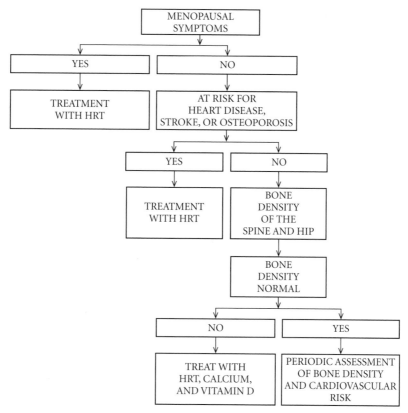

Figure 13.1 Flow diagram to help guide hormonal replacement therapy (HRT) for menopausal women. HRT involves the use of estrogen or progestin, or both, depending on the clinical situation (see text).

past the age when their bone mass is at its peak. Until she reaches the age of about 30 years, a woman's body forms more bone than is removed. Thereafter, bone loss is gradual until menopause, during the first 5 years of which it accelerates to nearly 4% or 5% a year and then slows down again.

In addition to menopause, other factors can increase the risk of bone loss and osteoporosis: a low-calcium diet, race (white and Asian women have a higher incidence), lack of exercise, small or thin body frame, family history, and alcohol and tobacco use. In addition, certain medications, such as corticosteroids and diuretics (water pills), can promote bone loss and osteoporosis. Women with epilepsy may have an additional risk factor for osteoporosis. Some antiepileptic medications may be associated with mineral loss from bone, osteoporosis, and similar problems. This issue is addressed in detail in Chapter 16.

Osteoporosis can be treated, but it is better to take preventive measures. A diet high in calcium, calcium supplements, and vitamin D have been shown to prevent excessive bone loss. In addition, physical exercise increases bone mass before menopause and slows bone loss after menopause. HRT with estrogen also prevents osteoporosis and is a major reason for menopausal women to consider HRT (Fig. 13.1). Avoiding alcohol and cigarette smoking is also beneficial. Because some antiepileptic medications have been associated with impaired bone mineralization, women taking such drugs should assess their overall risk of osteoporosis with their physician and take appropriate measures (see Chapter 16). Bone-density measurements can help women to determine whether they have sustained excessive bone loss (Fig. 13.1).

Other effects of menopause

Vaginal and urinary tract symptoms can occur as a consequence of menopause. Low estrogen levels can cause vaginal dryness and irritation that may lead to itching and sometimes pain, especially during sexual intercourse. Menopause, however, does not have to interfere with a woman's sex life. Most women can continue to enjoy sexually active lives with the aid of vaginal lubricants or HRT with estrogen.

Menopause may also contribute to urinary problems such as frequent urination and an increased risk for urinary tract infections. HRT can also help these symptoms.

Sleep disturbances and emotional problems can also be a troubling part of menopause. Difficulty sleeping and fatigue are reported by 30–40% of all postmenopausal women.

Effects of menopause on women with epilepsy and seizures

To assess the potential influences of menopause on women with epilepsy and seizures we need to consider several issues: (1) the effect of menopause on the frequency and severity of seizures; (2) the possibility that antiepileptic medications will complicate menopause; and (3) whether HRT during menopause is appropriate for women with epilepsy. What follows is a discussion of each of these issues.

Effect of menopause on seizures

There is considerable evidence that female sex hormones and their fluctuations can influence seizures in women with epilepsy. How the hormonal changes of pregnancy, the menstrual cycle, and oral contraceptive therapy affect epileptic seizures is discussed in other chapters in this book. Although the influence of female hormones such as estrogen and progesterone on seizures is a highly complex issue, the prevalent view is that estrogen may increase the tendency for seizures, whereas progesterone appears to make seizures less likely.

Because menopause is characterized by a decrease in estrogen, one might expect the risk of seizures to decrease at this time. However, the situation is probably much more complex because progesterone levels also decrease. Other hormonal, endocrine, and metabolic changes that occur during menopause can also influence the risk of seizures. It is, therefore, difficult to predict exactly what any individual woman with epilepsy should expect during or after menopause. It is the complex interaction of all these various factors combined with a woman's own individual characteristics and sensitivities that ultimately determines the effect menopause will have on her seizures.

However, despite the fact that it is not currently possible to predict exactly how menopause will affect any individual woman with epilepsy, some recent studies offer some helpful guidelines. For example, in a study of our own comparing menopausal women with epilepsy to younger premenopausal women who also had seizures, we found that seizures were similar in frequency and severity in both groups.

However, some of the menopausal women reported that menopause did seem to influence their seizures. Among the approximately 60 women we interviewed with epilepsy preceding their menopause, the majority (60%) reported that their seizures did not change in frequency or improved with the onset of their menopause. Indeed, about 30% of patients in this group actually reported some improvement in their seizures with menopause. However, approximately 40% of these patients noted that their seizures worsened in menopause.

Our results are similar to those of a previous study in Poland that described a somewhat smaller group of menopausal women. In that study, the majority of women (70%) described no change or improvement in their seizures with menopause (50% describing no change and 20% noting improvement). This Polish study also found that seizures worsened for about 30% of women, somewhat less than in our study. Such figures are reassuring in that most women with epilepsy (60–70%) described no change or improvement in their seizures with menopause. However, it is also important to note that 30–40% reported some worsening, a concerning figure warranting attention. If such a high proportion of menopausal women with epilepsy do experience worsening of their seizures, specific treatment strategies may need to be developed for these women.

One unforeseen finding in our study was that about one-fifth of the menopausal women we interviewed first experienced seizures during menopause. This is not entirely surprising because it is well known that seizures and epilepsy can start in later years as a consequence of concomitant illnesses such as strokes, brain tumors, and Alzheimer's disease. Some of the women in our study were older and the onset of their seizures was related to this type of illness. However, other women who had seizures beginning closer to the start of menopause lacked a clear etiology for their epilepsy. This observation, although still preliminary, raises the possibility that some women going through menopause may be at greater risk for developing epilepsy. Further studies need to be done to confirm this observation.

Antiepileptic medications in menopause

Older patients with epilepsy have special problems with medications in general and antiepileptic medications in particular. These older patients are especially sensitive to the sedating and potentially adverse cognitive effects of medications such as antiepileptic drugs and may have more medical problems requiring medications that can interact with their antiepileptic drugs. Some antiepileptics may therefore not work as expected, or could produce unanticipated toxic reactions.

There are some medication interactions of particular concern for menopausal women, most importantly the possible interaction between antiepileptic medications and HRT with estrogen. The effects of estrogen on antiepileptic medications vary depending on the drug, but can be significant.

In addition, antiepileptic medications may influence the effectiveness of HRT or cause problems for women taking oral contraceptives (Chapter 18). It is known that some antiepileptic medications decrease the effectiveness of such birth control measures. Similar interactions between hormonal treatments and antiepileptic medications may impair the effectiveness of HRT in menopause. Calcium supplements, which are often prescribed for osteoporosis, can also decrease the absorption of some antiepileptic medications. Women should discuss these potential interactions with their physicians. Blood tests to determine precise levels of antiepileptic medications present in a woman's body may help to define how these interactions affect an individual's medication metabolism and to plan optimal strategies for treatment.

Older individuals may experience metabolic changes that influence antiepileptic drug metabolism: decrease in liver function, kidney function, gastrointestinal absorption, and relative amounts of body muscle compared to fat. Such changes can all influence antiepileptic blood levels, causing problems such as drug toxicity or poor seizure control. Menopausal women should consider all of these changes if unexplained problems with antiepileptic drug treatment occur.

Hormone replacement therapy in menopause

For a menopausal woman, whether or not she has epilepsy, the decision to use HRT can be difficult. There are several important issues to consider (Fig. 13.1). HRT with estrogen can be very beneficial because it effectively treats many of the adverse symptoms of menopause (see Table 13.1). For example, it can decrease the risk of cardiovascular disease and osteoporosis, both very serious problems for menopausal women. HRT is not without some risk, however. One clear risk is that estrogen can increase a woman's chances of developing uterine cancer, an issue only for women who have not had a hysterectomy. Fortunately, this risk can be avoided if menopausal women who have not had hysterectomies take both estrogen and progesterone (Fig. 13.1). However, women taking this combination of hormones usually experience a recurrence of monthly uterine bleeding, which some find undesirable.

Another concern for menopausal women is the potential for HRT to increase the risk of breast cancer. To date, evidence for this increased risk has not been conclusive, but the risk varies and women at higher risk for breast cancer, such as women with a family history of breast cancer, should be particularly cautious. Each woman should discuss with her physician the risks and the benefits of HRT to arrive at the best treatment plan for her individual situation.

For the woman with epilepsy, HRT with estrogen poses another problem because it can influence antiepileptic metabolism and seizures. In fact, some physicians may be reluctant to prescribe HRT to women with epilepsy because of concern that it could worsen seizures. However, there is no convincing evidence to support that view. Moreover, given the tremendous potential benefits of HRT for menopausal women in terms of preventing cardiovascular disease and osteoporosis, and alleviating other menopausal symptoms, menopausal women with epilepsy should not be deprived of the benefits of HRT because of unproven concerns that it many worsen their seizures.

In fact, our own limited observations of the menopausal women in our study do not indicate that HRT is likely to affect adversely menopausal women with epilepsy. Most women in our studies noted no significant worsening in their seizures when receiving HRT. Of the menopausal women we interviewed, about 30 had some experience with HRT for menopause. Of these women, over two-thirds noted no change in their seizures while on HRT. Of the remaining one-third, about half reported improvement in their seizures and half described some worsening. These preliminary observations suggest no major ill-effects of HRT in menopausal women with epilepsy. However, each patient must be considered individually and menopausal women who do experience worsening of their seizures with HRT should consult their physicians to determine how best to manage the problem. Based on existing evidence and our own preliminary observations, withholding HRT from menopausal women with epilepsy because of concern that it may worsen their seizures is unwarranted.

A recommended approach to the decision-making process for HRT in menopause is outlined in Figure 13.1. This is a useful guide for all menopausal women, and women with epilepsy can use it as well because the presence of seizures is not a contraindication to HRT. However, the effects of HRT should be monitored in women with epilepsy and treatment should be adjusted as necessary.

SELECTED REFERENCES

Abbasi F, Krumholz A, Kittner SJ, Langenburg P. Effects of menopause on women with epilepsy. *Epilepsia* 1995; 36 (Suppl. 4):148 (abstract).

Abbasi F, Krumholz A, Kittner SJ, Langenburg P. New onset epilepsy in older women is influenced by menopause. *Epilepsia* 1996; 37 (Suppl. 5):97 (abstract).

Herzog AG. Reproductive endocrine considerations and hormonal therapy for women with epilepsy. *Epilepsia* 1991; 32(Suppl. 6):S27–S33.

Mattson RH. Use of oral contraceptives by women with epilepsy. *J Am Med Assoc* 1986; 256:238–40.

Morrell MJ. Hormones and epilepsy through the lifetime. *Epilepsia* 1992; 33 (Suppl. 4):549–61.

Rosciszeweska D. Epilepsy and menstruation. In *Epilepsy*, ed. A Hopkins. Chapman and Hall, London, 1987, 373–81.

Thacker HL. Current issues in menopausal hormone replacement therapy. *Cleveland Clin J* 1996; 63:344–53.

Part IV

Health challenges for women with epilepsy

14

Reproductive health for women with epilepsy

Martha J. Morrell

Women with epilepsy are less likely to have children than women without epilepsy. For many years, it was assumed this was because women with epilepsy were less likely to be married and, when married, more likely to choose to remain childless. Women with epilepsy now have marriage rates equivalent to women without epilepsy. Better prenatal care and information about the excellent outcome for more than 90% of pregnancies in women with epilepsy suggest that more women are able to choose to be mothers. However, birth rates remain lower than expected. In part, this can be explained by recent findings that women with epilepsy are less likely to ovulate and more likely to have disorders of reproductive hormones. Whether these reproductive health disturbances are caused by seizures, by antiepileptic medications, or by both, is now being debated in the medical community. This chapter discusses some of the reproductive disturbances in women with epilepsy and points out signs and symptoms that women should report to their health-care providers.

MJM

Introduction

Having epilepsy often means more than having seizures. Other areas of health may also be negatively impacted in the person with epilepsy, including reproductive health. Medical research suggests that women with epilepsy are more likely to have irregular menstrual cycles, menstrual cycles during which ovulation does not occur, and disturbances in the hormones that regulate the menstrual cycle and are needed for normal fertility.

Reproductive health disturbances described in women with epilepsy include menstrual abnormalities such as amenorrhea (not menstruating), oligomenorrhea (menstrual cycle length greater than 35 days), and metrorrhagia (irregular menstrual cycle with excessive menstrual flow). One-third to one-half of women with epilepsy have menstrual disorders. Some women with epilepsy have polycystic ovaries, a condition in which there are multiple cysts on the ovaries, instead of the one large cyst from which the egg is released at ovulation.

Women with epilepsy may also have abnormalities in the amount (concentration) of hormones released from the pituitary gland of the brain, as well as in the rhythm of release of these hormones. Some of these pituitary hormones – follicle-stimulating hormone (FSH) and luteinizing hormone (LH) – act on the ovaries to regulate the menstrual cycle, ensure that ovulation occurs, and control the synthesis (manufacturing) and release of estrogen and progesterone, the female sex hormones. Disturbances in these pituitary hormones are associated with anovulation and with abnormalities in the length and regularity of the menstrual cycle.

Menstrual cycle abnormalities, polycystic ovaries, and disruption in pituitary and ovarian hormones may cause infertility (difficulty becoming pregnant or carrying a pregnancy to completion). Fertility, defined as the number of children born alive, is reduced in women with epilepsy. Some medical papers report that fertility rates in women with epilepsy are about 75% those of women without epilepsy. Another study found that women with epilepsy are only one-third as likely to conceive as their nonepileptic sisters. Reduced fertility appears to be a result of difficulty becoming pregnant as well as of higher rates of spontaneous abortion, miscarriage, and pregnancy complications. One study based in the Netherlands found that spontaneous abortions were almost twice as likely to occur in the pregnancies of women with epilepsy than in controls.

Scientists do not know whether these reproductive disturbances are caused by the seizures, by the antiepileptic medications used to control seizures, or perhaps even by both. In one study of reproductive function in women with epilepsy, reproductive dysfunctions were as frequent in women not treated with antiepileptic medications as in those who received antiepileptic drugs. However, other investigators believe that particular antiepileptic drugs may be more likely to be associated with menstrual disorders. In one study, menstrual disturbances were reported in 45% of women receiving valproate and in 19% of women receiving carbamazepine for epilepsy.

Antiepileptic drugs that alter the hepatic cytochrome P450 (CyP450) enzyme system can negatively affect reproductive function by changing the concentrations of hormones in the brain. Antiepileptic drugs that increase the activity of liver enzymes increase the breakdown (metabolism) of female sex hormones and also increase the rate at which the hormones attach to circulating proteins in the bloodstream. When hormones are attached to proteins, they are not able to cross from the bloodstream to the brain. This reduces the amount of hormone in the brain. Some research suggests that these reductions in brain hormones may cause symptoms such as reduced sexual desire and difficulty with sexual arousal. The medication valproate inhibits these liver enzymes and decreases the breakdown of androgens. Some women on valproate have an increase in the male-type hormone testosterone. This may be associated with abnormal menstrual cycle length and regularity, and with a change in the distribution of body hair and thinning of scalp hair. Some of the newer antiepileptic medications, such as lamotrigine and gabapentin, do not cause a change in the levels of these hormones.

Reproductive disorders in women with epilepsy

Women with epilepsy appear to be at risk for anovulatory cycles, polycystic ovaries, and disturbance in the hypothalamic–pituitary axis – the system that regulates the menstrual cycle and ovarian production of female sex steroid hormones (see Fig. 11.2).

The menstrual cycle

At puberty, the female pattern of cyclic hypothalamic and pituitary hormone release occurs. After the first few menstrual cycles, most women have a regular cycle length of about 25–30 days.

In the beginning of the cycle, the pituitary hormone FSH is released in relatively large amounts. This hormone encourages the development of one primary 'egg' or follicle in the ovary. This stage of the menstrual cycle (the follicular phase) lasts approximately 14 days (although this time is variable).

Ovulation occurs next, when the pituitary releases a surge of LH, which causes the egg to be released from the ovary. The egg travels to the fallopian tube, then to the uterus. If the egg is fertilized with a male sperm, the fertilized egg (embryo) attaches to the thickened wall of the uterus. If the egg is not fertilized, implantation cannot occur and the uterine lining sloughs. This causes the menstrual flow.

During the first half of the cycle (the follicular phase), the hormone estrogen is released in steadily increasing amounts. With ovulation, there is a surge in estrogen, after which estrogen production drops until the beginning of the next menstrual cycle. When the egg is released from the ovary at ovulation, a structure is formed that is called the corpus luteum. The corpus luteum produces the hormone progesterone, which increases steadily over the second half of the menstrual cycle (the luteal phase). The luteal phase lasts approximately 14 days and there is less variability than with the follicular phase. If the egg is not fertilized, the corpus luteum stops producing progesterone. There is an abrupt fall in progesterone several days before menstrual flow begins.

In most women, ovulation will occur in about nine out of ten cycles. One out of ten menstrual cycles will be anovulatory. In an anovulatory cycle, the egg does not leave the ovary, a corpus luteum is not formed, and progesterone remains low during the luteal phase of the cycle.

As many as one-third of menstrual cycles are anovulatory in women with epilepsy. Anovulatory cycles may be signaled by longer than normal cycles, missed cycles, or mid-cycle menstrual bleeding. Researchers are now trying to determine the causes of anovulatory cycles in women with epilepsy. Possible causes include disruption in hypothalamic input to the pituitary, in release of pituitary hormones, or abnormal response of the ovary to the pituitary hormones. Scientists know that some women with epilepsy have disturbances in the release of hypothalamic and pituitary hormones. Recent work suggests that there may be a problem with the ovarian response as well.

Some women with epilepsy have polycystic ovaries and elevated levels of androgen hormones (testosterone) produced by the ovary. This affects 20–40% of women with epilepsy and appears to be most common for women receiving the antiepileptic drug valproate (Depakote).

The significance of these findings is not entirely understood, but polycystic ovaries and elevated testosterone are also seen in a condition called polycystic ovary syndrome. Polycystic ovary syndrome is the most common cause of infertility in women. It is a gynecological syndrome that affects about 15% of all women. Women with this condition may have increased body hair and scalp-hair thinning, obesity, and acne. Hormone abnormalities include increased testosterone and disturbances in pituitary hormones. The ovaries have multiple cysts, which can be imaged by an ultrasound test. Infertility is one consequence of this condition, because of frequent anovulatory menstrual cycles. An abnormality in the insulin receptor causes abnormal uptake of glucose (sugar) into cells. As a result of this insulin abnormality, women with this syndrome are at greater risk for diabetes. Other health risks associated with polycystic ovary syndrome are endometrial cancer and cardiovascular disease. When detected, gynecologists usually elect to treat the affected woman with hormones, diet, and exercise.

Whether the polycystic ovaries, increased testosterone, and higher frequency of anovulatory cycles in women with epilepsy are the same as polycystic ovary syndrome is not known. Therefore, we do not know whether women with epilepsy and polycystic ovaries have the same health risks as women with polycystic ovary syndrome. However, if women with epilepsy have any signs of polycystic ovary syndrome (menstrual cycles shorter than 23 days or longer than 35 days, mid-cycle spotting, a change in body or scalp hair, acne, or obesity), an evaluation should be conducted to check for hormone abnormalities and to image the ovaries with an ultrasound examination.

We do not know what causes polycystic ovaries, anovulatory cycles, and elevated testosterone in some women with epilepsy. Electrical epileptic discharges in the brain may alter pituitary hormones and abnormally stimulate the ovaries. Changes in ovarian hormones caused by antiepileptic drug interactions could also cause anovulatory cycles. Finally, the antiepileptic drug valproate may specifically increase the risk.

Until we know exactly what is causing reproductive cycle disturbances in women with epilepsy, what should a woman do? First, be alert for the following signs and symptoms:

- a menstrual cycle length that varies by more than 5 days from the first day of menstrual bleeding to the first day of menstrual bleeding of the next cycle,
- a menstrual cycle that is shorter than 23 days or longer than 35 days,
- mid-cycle menstrual spotting,
- weight gain,
- increase in body hair or thinning of scalp hair,
- acne,
- reduced sexual interest or difficulty becoming sexually aroused.

These signs and symptoms may indicate that menstrual cycles are anovulatory and/or that there is a hormonal disturbance. Bring this information to the attention of your neurologist and gynecologist, who will arrange for the appropriate additional evaluation.

Conclusion

Reproductive disorders create great challenges for women with epilepsy. With better understanding of the types of reproductive problems that can occur in women with epilepsy and why they occur, concerned women and their health-care providers can arrange for appropriate testing if a reproductive disorder is suspected, and treatment can be offered if a reproductive disorder is found. Antiepileptic medication choice will take into account seizure control, tolerability, and preservation of reproductive health. In the meantime, health-care providers and consumers require better access to information about the reproductive health issues faced by women with epilepsy.

SELECTED REFERENCES

Isojarvi JIT, Laatikainen TJ, Pakarinen AJ, Juntunen KTS, Myllyla VV. Polycystic ovaries and hyperandrogenism in women taking valproate for epilepsy. *N Engl J Med* 1993; 329:1383–8.

Morrell MJ. Hormones and epilepsy through the lifetime. *Epilepsia* 1992; 33(S4):49–61.

Morrell MJ. Effects of epilepsy on women's reproductive health. *Epilepsia* 1998; 39(S8): S32–7.

Zahn CA, Morrell MJ, Collins SD, Labiner DM, Yerby MS. Management issues for women with epilepsy: a review of the literature. American Academy of Neurology Practice Guidelines. *Neurology* 1998; 51:949–56.

15

Sexual dysfunction in epilepsy

Martha J. Morrell

Shortly after I became a specialist in the care of people with epilepsy, I realized that many of my patients were not happy with their sexuality. Women and men reported to me that they had less sexual desire than they wished they had. Men complained of difficulty achieving erections and women noted painful, difficult intercourse. In going to the medical literature, I found many reports that sexual dysfunction was common in people with epilepsy, but did not find good explanations as to why this should be. I had done research into sexual function earlier in my career and decided that there was a real need for research in sexuality in people with epilepsy. Our research team is still working in this area. We have learned a lot, but there is more to know. We find that about one-third of people with epilepsy have less interest in sex than they would like and about 40% have physical sexual problems. These physical problems affect sexual arousal, making intercourse difficult and not as pleasant. Fortunately, there are effective treatments for the kind of sexual problems that arise with epilepsy – but sexual symptoms have to be identified and discussed. Physicians and patients usually do not discuss sexuality. However, even if it is a little hard to begin the discussion, sexual symptoms are important. The health-care provider will be glad the topic is brought up so that an appropriate medical evaluation can be completed and helpful treatment can begin.

MJM

Sexuality is a very private, but extremely important, part of most people's life. Many medical and neurological conditions – including epilepsy – can negatively affect sexuality. This chapter discusses some of the sexual symptoms experienced by some people with epilepsy and reviews appropriate diagnostic tests and treatments. However, in order to understand why sexual life might be impacted by epilepsy, it is helpful first to discuss the biology of sexuality.

Most scientists think of sexuality as comprised of two main components: sexual desire and physiological sexual arousal. Sexual desire refers to sexual

Figure 15.1 Primary components of sexuality.

interest, or libido. It depends on a person's emotional and psychological well-being and also requires an appropriate sexual stimulus. Physiological sexual arousal refers to stereotyped events that occur in the body when people are in a sexually exciting situation. Physiological sexual arousal is also called potency. In a man, this is evident by a penile erection and by ejaculation. The same events occur in women, although physiological sexual arousal in women is not so visually obvious (Fig. 15.1).

Normal sexuality depends not only on emotions, but also on biology. To have healthy sexual feelings and responses, certain regions of the brain, specifically the frontal and temporal lobes, must function normally. In addition, hormones of the pituitary gland and of the ovaries or testes must be present in adequate amounts. The spinal cord must also function normally, as must the nerves that travel from the spinal cord to genital tissues and the genital structures – the penis in the man and the vagina in the woman.

Animal studies have shown that certain areas of the brain are important in supporting normal sexual desire and responsiveness. These include the temporal lobe, particularly the limbic structures contained within the temporal lobe, and the frontal lobe (Fig. 15.2). When electrical stimulation is applied to the temporal lobe of monkeys, penile erections occur. When these structures are destroyed by electricity or chemicals, the animal is unable to have an erection. Erectile failure also occurs with lesions in certain areas of the frontal lobe, particularly the medial and deep areas, called the orbital frontal cortex.

Hormones are also important for normal sexuality. The hypothalamus in the brain releases a trophic hormone called gonadotropin-releasing hormone (GnRH). This hormone acts on the pituitary gland of the brain to stimulate the release of luteinizing hormone (LH) and follicle-stimulating hormone (FSH). These two hormones act on the ovaries in women to

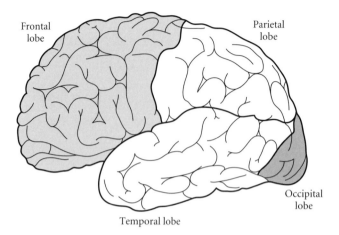

Figure 15.2 Areas of the brain important for normal sexual desire and responsiveness.

stimulate the release of estrogen and progesterone and on the testes in men to stimulate the release of testosterone. These testicular and ovarian hormones are called sex steroid hormones. The sex steroid hormones then travel back to the brain and act both to stimulate and to inhibit the release of hormones of the hypothalamus and the pituitary. In nonhuman animals, GnRH and LH are important for normal sexual behavior. The sex steroid hormones maintain secondary sexual characteristics. That means that testosterone causes male hair growth and other features that are typical of a male, whereas estrogen and progesterone promote female-type hair growth, breast enlargement, and other features typical of females. Sufficient amounts of testosterone and other testosterone-like hormones (androgens) must be present in men for them to have normal sexual desire and to be able to achieve normal sexual physiological arousal. In women, estrogen is important to maintain normal physiological sexual arousal. Recent evidence suggests that androgens are important in women in order for them to maintain normal sexual desire (Fig. 15.3).

The physiological sexual response is stereotyped in men and women. This was first described by Masters and Johnson in 1966 and has since been confirmed by others (Fig. 15.4). The first phase of physiological sexual arousal is excitement. In the excitement phase, blood is shifted to genital tissues, which gradually become engorged. In men, this is evident as an erection. The same

Sex Steroids Support Sex Behavior

	desire	arousal
male	androgens	androgens
female	androgens	estrogens

Figure 15.3 Types of hormones linked to desire and arousal.

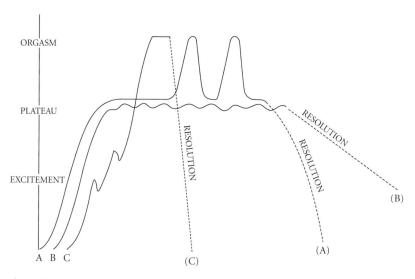

Figure 15.4 Physiological sexual response in men and women.

phenomena occur in women within the vagina. In addition, the heart rate and breathing rate increase and perspiration may occur. When vasocongestion in genital tissues is maximal, the plateau phase begins. At this point, the man has achieved a maximal erection. The plateau phase is variable in length and terminated when orgasm occurs. Orgasm in men and women is remarkably similar. It is characterized by 0.8 per second rhythmic contractions of muscles of the genital tissues and the pelvis floor. In women, this includes rhythmic contractions of the uterus and the fallopian tubes. Physiological sexual arousal requires that nerves going from the spinal cord to the genital tissues be working normally. The nerves of both the sympathetic nervous system and the somatic nervous system are utilized. Following orgasm, there is a refractory period, during which no amount of sexual stimulation can cause excitement. The refractory period is longer in men than in women, which is why women are capable of having multiple orgasms.

Problems with sexuality in people with epilepsy have been described for many years. Scientists writing in this field have observed that men and women with epilepsy are likely to have diminished sexual desire and problems with sexual arousal. Between one-third and two-thirds of men and women with seizure disorders may find that their sexual desire is less than they would wish. Approximately one-third of men with epilepsy may have occasional problems with erections and men and women with epilepsy have been reported to have a higher incidence of orgasm failure. However, most of these studies were performed in men and women with uncontrolled seizures who required multiple antiepileptic drugs (AEDs.)

In a study at the Stanford Comprehensive Epilepsy Center, women with epilepsy were evaluated. These women in general had well-controlled seizures and were taking only one AED. In this study, sexual desire appeared to be normal, as did the ability to achieve orgasm. However, women with epilepsy complained of painful intercourse because of vaginal dryness and difficulty relaxing muscles at the entrance of the vagina. This caused pain with insertion of the penis. This complaint arose in about one out of every three women with epilepsy. In addition, approximately one-third said that they were not satisfied with their overall sexual function.

Further analysis revealed that women with epilepsy were somewhat less likely to be aroused in specific sexual situations. However, a more striking finding was that sexual activity created more anxiety for women with epilepsy then for women without epilepsy. It may be that seizures are sometimes associated with sexual feelings. If that were the case, sexual feelings would become negatively associated with seizures and would obviously be much less enjoyable. Also, many individuals find that their seizures are more likely to occur when they hyperventilate or engage in strenuous exercise, both of which can be a part of sexual activity.

Men with epilepsy may also have problems with sexual function. In the community, erectile dysfunction is thought to be a problem for less than 15% of men. However, men with epilepsy may have a higher rate of impotence, perhaps as high as 58% in those with seizures that are not controlled. In order to understand why impotence occurs, it is helpful to sort out whether it is psychological or physiological. To do this, tests can be conducted to see whether erections occur in the daytime or nighttime. If erections are impaired during the daytime but not at night, it is likely that the impotence has a psychological basis. However, if a man is also lacking spontaneous erections during sleep, it is likely that the erectile difficulty is due to physiological or biological problems. Several studies suggest that men with epilepsy lack the normal erections that occur approximately three times a night while asleep. This implies that men with epilepsy who have problems with impotence have a physiological, not an emotional, problem.

Recording erections during sleep does not reproduce a normal sexual situation. In order to understand how men and women with epilepsy would react in a situation that more closely resembles a normal sexual encounter, we performed a study. Men and women with epilepsy arising from the temporal lobe of the brain were evaluated, as well as men and women without epilepsy who were of similar age. In this study, subjects volunteered to watch a series of videotapes, some of which were erotic. While the videotapes were shown, noninvasive devices that were put in place by the people participating in the study measured blood flow in the penis and vagina (Fig. 15.5). The men and women with temporal lobe epilepsy had less blood flow to genital tissues in response to the erotic films than did the men and women without epilepsy. This suggests that the first phase of biological sexual arousal is altered by the condition of epilepsy. This is further evidence that sexual problems in

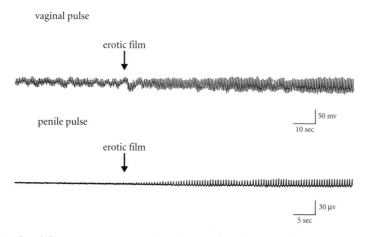

Figure 15.5 Blood flow measurements in male and female genitalia in response to erotic film.

men and women with epilepsy are not psychological but are related to some physiological disturbance. Of note, in this particular study, men and women were asked to rate how sexually aroused they *felt* when they watched the erotic videotapes. They described themselves as quite aroused. Therefore, the lack of physiological arousal was not noticeable to the study participants themselves.

From our studies, we believe that men and women with epilepsy may be more likely to have problems with physiological or biological arousal. Women with epilepsy may have pain with sexual intercourse and men with epilepsy may be more likely to have difficulties achieving an erection or in ejaculation. However, for most women and men with epilepsy, sexual experience and desire are normal.

Scientists are investigating the cause of sexual problems in men and women with epilepsy and there is likely to be more than one possible cause. Normal sexuality requires positive self-esteem, secure sexual identity, and the opportunity to engage in sexual activity. People with epilepsy may have poor self-esteem because of seizures and, perhaps, as a result of side effects of AEDs. Certainly, some individuals with epilepsy experience social prejudice. Particularly in adolescence, individuals with seizures may be treated unfairly – especially if seizures occur in school or the work place. In addition, poor self-perception will also contribute to restricted social opportunities. Individuals with low self-esteem may not actively seek out social situations, fearing that they will not be accepted.

Scientists evaluating sexual function and other social abilities in individuals with chronic illness find that disease acceptance plays an important role. For individuals with diabetes, hypertension, and other chronic illnesses, a realistic acceptance of the disease enhances all social behaviors. Good disease acceptance implies that the individual realistically understands the limitations imposed upon her or him by the disease – neither minimizing nor exaggerating its impact. Individuals who underestimate or overestimate the effects of any illness on their life do not have good disease acceptance. This may lead to excessive restrictions, in the case of overestimation of disease severity, or unrealistic expectations of normality, when the disease impact is denied or ignored. Disease acceptance has also been shown to influence sexual function in individuals with neurological illness. In one study in Scandinavia (Jensen, 1992), when individuals had good disease acceptance, sexual function was more likely to be satisfactory. It is also important that the sexual partner has good disease acceptance, as any unrealistic attitudes on the part of the partner will impact sexual interactions as well.

For many years, it was felt that most sexual dysfunction in epilepsy could be attributed to poor social interactions. In our research at Stanford, we did not find this to be so. In our population of patients coming to the Stanford Comprehensive Epilepsy Center, men and women surveyed had as much (actually more) sexual experience than did healthy college students upon which the inventory was based. Also, sexual attitudes were largely unaffected by epilepsy. Individuals described themselves as interested in sex and imagined that they would be aroused in a number of hypothetical sexual situations.

Disruption to areas of the brain controlling sexual behavior may also cause sexual dysfunction. Epileptic discharges may cause such brain dysfunction, particularly if the epileptic discharges occur in regions of the brain in which sexuality is located, including the frontal and temporal lobes. Lesions in the mesial frontal lobe and in the hippocampus of the temporal lobe, as well as in connecting structures, cause sexual dysfunction in animals. Electrical stimulation applied to many of these areas may stimulate sexual behavior. Stimulation of the orbitofrontal gyrus in the frontal lobe causes erections in male rodents, whereas destructive lesions in this region can impair erections.

Destructive brain lesions may occur as a result of head trauma, stroke, developmental abnormalities, infection, abnormal blood vessels, or foreign tissue lesions such as brain tumors. These lesions may be the trigger for epilepsy and may independently impair the normal function of these brain regions, including normal sexual function. Seizure discharges may also cause a disturbance. Some authors believe that sexual dysfunction is more likely to occur when seizures are very frequent. It has been observed that sexual dysfunction is likely to occur at the time that seizures arise and that seizure control, whether by medication or by epilepsy surgery, often results in improved sexuality.

Epilepsy may lead to disturbances in the hormones that support sexual behavior. These include the pituitary hormones, LH and FSH, as well as prolactin. Although a role for FSH in sexual behavior has not been demonstrated in humans, in animals this hormone is important to maintain normal sexuality. LH stimulates sexual behavior. Lack of this hormone results in an animal that is uninterested in sex and is physiologically less able to respond sexually. Prolactin excess is a common cause of impotence in nonepileptic men. Elevations in prolactin caused by repeated seizures may also cause sexual dysfunction, including reduced desire, and erectile difficulties.

Testosterone is also important to maintain normal sexual desire in women. Ordinarily, this testosterone is derived from the conversion of estrogen from the ovaries by metabolic processes. Low levels of estrogen and progesterone in men and women with epilepsy may be part of the cause of difficulties with sexual desire and sexual arousal.

AEDs also contribute to sexual dysfunction. They exert their anti-seizure effects by depressing the excitability of brain nerve cells (neurons). Unfortunately, the AEDs act on all neurons of the cerebral cortex, not just the epileptic neurons. Therefore, neuronal function may be depressed diffusely. This translates into feelings of mental slowing and other common side effects of AEDs, such as difficulty with vision focus and problems with coordination and balance. Fortunately, these side effects, if they occur, are usually minor. However, some individuals may be particularly sensitive to the effects of an AED and have persistent problems with side effects, which limit that drug's usefulness. In one study of phenytoin (Dilantin), carbamazepine (Tegretol), primidone (Mysoline), and phenobarbital, it was noted that as many as 20% of men developed erectile difficulties occasionally or chronically as each medication was begun. This was most likely to occur with phenobarbital. Detailed studies of the effects of AEDs on individual sexual functioning have not been performed. However, in the course of practice, most physicians caring for people with epilepsy have noticed that some people will develop sexual symptoms on a specific AED and will be asymptomatic on another.

AEDs may also affect sexuality by influencing the hormones important for maintaining sexual behavior, as discussed above. AEDs that increase the activity of liver enzymes (carbamazepine, phenytoin, and phenobarbital) increase the breakdown of sex steroid hormones. This lowers the effective level of the hormones and may cause a mild hormone deficiency.

Most sexual disorders are treatable. The first step is to bring any sexual problems to the attention of your physician, who will conduct an examination to make sure that other medical conditions can be excluded (Table 15.1). Other medical conditions that can cause problems with sexuality include high blood pressure, diabetes mellitus, spinal cord disease, and hormonal

Table 15.1. Causes of sexual dysfunction

Drugs	
Psychotropic drugs	Monoamine oxidase inhibitors, phenothiazines, barbiturates, benodiazepines, alcohol
Antihypertensive drugs	Methyldopa, β-blockers, α-adrenergic blockers
Other	Anticholinergics, stimulants, narcotics
Medical	
Vascular	Small-vessel disease secondary to diabetes, hypertension, hyperlipidemia
Endocrine	Hyperprolactinemia, hypothyroidism or hyperthyroidism, significantly low testosterone
Systemic illness	Renal, hepatic, cardiac, or pulmonary; cancer
Urogenital	Infections, injury
Neurological	
Spinal cord	Injury or disease
Neuropathy	Peripheral, autonomic
Cortical lesions	Frontal lobe, temporal lobe
Psychogenic	
Psychiatric	Psychosis, depression, bipolar illness
Intrapsychiatric	Result of religious, social, family taboos; early-life sexual experience, low self-esteem
Extrapsychic	Dysfunctional relationship

abnormalities such as thyroid disease. A thorough physical examination will be performed and laboratory tests will be obtained, which will include a complete blood count, electrolyte panel, liver function tests, cholesterol, thyroid hormones, and pituitary and steroid hormone levels. For women, a complete gynecological examination should be conducted, including an internal exam (pelvic exam) and external evaluation. Infections of the uterus or cervix can contribute to sexual dysfunction, as can other physical abnormalities of genital tissues. For men, urological examination may include urodynamics and penile tumescence studies in order to determine whether the blood vessels and nerve cells to the penis are functioning normally.

If the physician has excluded other causes of sexual dysfunction, the dysfunction is probably related to epilepsy. If another medication can be substituted that will achieve good seizure control, that should be considered. Some individuals will be very symptomatic on one AED and completely free of symptoms on another. If seizures are not controlled, every effort should be made to achieve control, either by changing medication or by increasing the dosage of the medication already administered.

Specific therapies can be directed toward specific sexual problems. If women are experiencing vaginal dryness and consequent pain, a lubricating substance such as Astroglide or KY jelly may be helpful. Other products are available to increase vaginal moistness (such as Replense). Painful intercourse may also be due to muscle tightness, which can be corrected by practicing relaxation techniques. In extreme cases, gynecologists may use other techniques to stretch the muscles at the opening of the vagina.

There are many treatments for erectile difficulties. Biofeedback may be helpful. Medications such as yohimbine (Yocoon) can be taken orally and other medications (poparavine) can be injected in order to stimulate erections. There has been a great deal of interest in a medication called Viagra, which is helpful for men with impotence problems. (It is not known whether the medication can be helpful in women.) In more severe cases of impotence, penile implants may be surgically placed.

Counseling can often help women with sexual dysfunction. Relationship difficulties may cause sexual dysfunction and certainly may occur as a result of any problems with sexual interactions. Therefore, for most couples experiencing sexual difficulties, counseling is recommended in addition to the treatments mentioned above. This may take the form of marital or relationship counseling, or may be specific sexual therapy. In sexual therapy, couples practice sexual exercises according to a schedule established by the therapist.

Summary

Sexual dysfunction may arise in as many as one-third to one-half of men and women with epilepsy. The dysfunction appears to occur because of disruption to the brain regions controlling sexual behavior, disturbance of the hormones supporting sexual behavior, and the effects of AEDs. Although problems with sexual desire may occur, it is more likely that men or women with epilepsy will experience difficulty with sexual arousal. In a woman, this may include painful intercourse because of lack of lubrication and excessive tightness. In a man, it may involve difficulty achieving and maintaining an erection.

Help for sexual problems can be given if these difficulties are brought to the attention of a knowledgeable physician, which may be a neurologist, gynecologist, urologist, or internal medicine physician. An appropriate diagnostic evaluation will exclude other causes of sexual dysfunction. Treatment will then focus on seizure control, including alternative medications and the provision of directed therapies, which may include biofeedback, behavioral medicine techniques, newer medications to improve physiological sexual arousal, and more traditional couple or individual counseling.

New research is underway to define more clearly the types of sexual dysfunction occurring in individuals with epilepsy in order that more effective treatments can be devised. In the meantime, physicians treating people with epilepsy are increasingly recognizing this as a serious concern and are willing to work with their patients to find the best solution.

SELECTED REFERENCES

Jensen SB. Sexuality and chronic illness: biopsychological approach. *Semin Neurol* 1992; 12:135–40.

Levine SB. *Sexual Life. A Clinician's Guide*. Plenum Press, New York, 1992.

Masters WH, Johnson VE. *Human Sexual Response*. Little, Brown, Boston, 1966.

Morrell MJ. Sexuality in epilepsy. In *Epilepsy: a Comprehensive Textbook*, ed. J Engel, TA Pedley. Lippincott-Raven, Philadelphia, 1997, pp. 2021–6.

16

Bone health in women with epilepsy

Robert Marcus

Women are at greater risk for osteoporosis than men. For some years, physicians have been concerned that women with epilepsy are at particular risk for this condition, which is associated with bone fractures. Osteoporosis (thinning of the bones) may be caused by some antiepileptic drugs. Unfortunately, the available scientific information cannot tell health-care providers which medications cause bone disease and which of the drugs may be safer to use.

Dr Robert Marcus is a bone specialist who is an expert in bone health in women with epilepsy. He is a former Professor of Internal Medicine and Endocrinology at Stanford University. We have collaborated in a study evaluating bone density and bone turnover in women with epilepsy. This study, when it is complete, promises to provide helpful information about the effect of particular antiepileptic drugs on bone.

In the meantime, we recommend that all women with epilepsy employ good bone health practices; that is, regular, gravity-resisting exercise, good nutrition, and adequate calcium and vitamin D intake. Women with epilepsy should also have their bone density checked at least at menopause, if not earlier. More bone health recommendations will come out of the research being conducted.

MJM

Some people with epilepsy have an increased risk for a condition of the skeleton called osteoporosis. The purpose of this chapter is to clarify the nature of this relationship, to outline its possible causes, and to discuss current approaches to treatment.

Achieving and maintaining a healthy skeleton is determined largely by a person's genetic endowment (their genes), operating under the influence of numerous factors, including proper diet, regular physical activity, and adequate production of the female and male reproductive hormones estrogen and testosterone. When these factors are optimal, the skeleton develops adequate strength to withstand the demands of day-to-day weight-bearing and even extreme physical activities. If one or more of these factors is inadequate, deficits in the amount and quality of bone appear, leading to an increased risk for fractures, even in the absence of serious trauma. Such fractures are called fragility fractures. Osteoporosis is a condition in which the amount of bone is reduced and there is disruption of its normal microscopic appearance. When deficiencies of diet, activity, or hormone concentrations occur as an adult, bone loss ensues. When such deficiencies take place in a growing child, bone acquisition suffers, so that an individual enters adult life with a deficit in bone that is referred to as a reduction in peak bone mass.

Illness also poses a challenge to the skeleton, and this can happen in several ways (Fig. 16.1). Some illnesses directly affect the skeleton, particularly if they are associated with fever, inflammation, and weight loss, that is, with *systemic* manifestations. The effects of other illnesses may be less direct. Treatment of some conditions may make it necessary to restrict the diet or physical activity in ways that jeopardize the skeleton. Finally, some disorders may themselves cause no harm to the skeleton, but require long-term treatment with medications that have toxic effects on bone. An important example of such a medication is found in a group of drugs related to cortisone.

The problem of osteoporosis in people with epilepsy has long been assumed to be related to antiepileptic medications. However, it is important to point out that other aspects in the lifestyle of children and adults with epilepsy may themselves contribute to deficits in bone acquisition and maintenance. It has already been pointed out that robust physical activity is an important stimulus to bone acquisition during growth. If children are subjected to restrictions in activity, the amount of bone laid down will be less than that of more active children. In addition, attempts to impose severe dietary restrictions on children (such as with the ketogenic diet) may lead to inadequate consumption of calories, protein, calcium, and phosphorus, all of which are essential for skeletal growth. The truth is that, to date, very little work has been done to assess the contribution of activity, diet, or other lifestyle aspects of children with epilepsy to bone health.

That being said, a relationship between bone abnormalities and the long-term use of antiepileptic medications has been recognized for several decades. Early on, only severely affected patients were identified, but, over the last decade, it has become clear that milder abnormalities may be common. These abnormalities have been related primarily to two types of antiepileptic

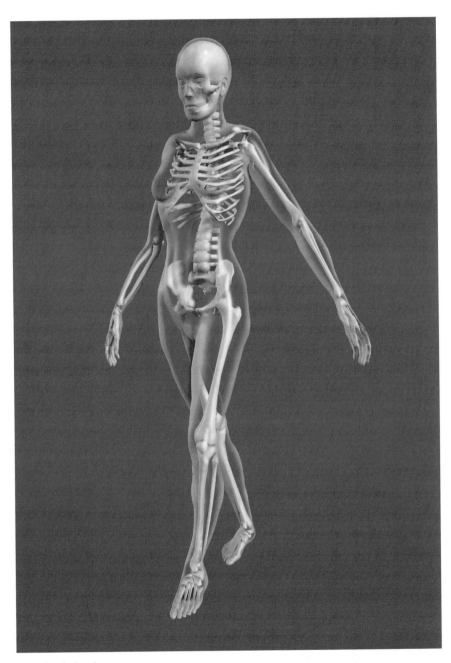

Figure 16.1 Female skeletal structure.

medication: hydantoins (which include phenytoin) and barbiturates (pheno-barbital and primedone). These drugs interact with the liver to stimulate an enzyme system (called the P450 enzymes) that depresses the production of active vitamin D. Hydantoins, in particular, also exert direct inhibitory effects on the intestine and on bone to interfere with the normal physiology of these tissues. The clinical severity of these abnormalities reflects the dose of medication as well as its duration of use.

Bone abnormalities have also been reported in adults and children receiving other antiepileptic medications, including carbamazepine (Tegretol, Carbatrol) and valproate (Depakote, Depakene). Scientists do not know how these medications might disrupt bone health. At this time, there is no information regarding the effects of the newer antiepileptic medications on bone.

Bone is not an inert structure like a column of marble. It is a living tissue that is constantly undergoing a process of breakdown and renewal called remodeling. Remodeling takes place in individual cycles, which are initiated by a group of cells called osteoclasts that dig a divot out of the bone. Different cells, called osteoblasts, fill in the holes by laying down new bone. The rate of bone remodeling is to some extent linked to the amount of calcium that comes into the bloodstream each day from the intestine. Under ordinary circumstances, roughly 30% of the calcium contained in the diet is absorbed into the blood. If dietary calcium intake decreases, or if there is impairment in the efficiency of calcium absorption, blood calcium concentration undergoes a slight reduction. Because the concentration of calcium in body fluids is so important to the normal functioning of the heart, muscles, nerves, and other body organs, a mechanism has evolved to protect against such reductions in blood calcium. This protective mechanism involves glands in the neck called the parathyroid glands, which produce a hormone called parathyroid hormone (PTH). This hormone travels in the circulation to the kidney, where it stimulates the conservation of calcium and reduces urinary calcium loss, and also to the bone, where it stimulates an increase in bone remodeling that delivers more calcium to the blood. Unfortunately, bone remodeling is itself not a completely efficient process, so that a little bit of bone is lost when each bone remodeling event is finished.

As stated above, antiepileptic drugs of the barbiturate and hydantoin type modestly impair the liver's ability to manufacture an active form of vitamin D.

Table 16.1. Recommendations to maintain good bone health

✓ Make certain that calcium intake is adequate
  ○ Before puberty   1500 mg per day
  ○ After puberty   1000 mg per day
  ○ While pregnant   1500 mg per day
  ○ Menopause   1500 mg per day
✓ Take additional vitamin D (400 units)
✓ Do gravity-resisting exercise for at least 20 minutes (running, brisk walking, weight lifting, ball sports, for example)
✓ If postmenopausal, discuss with your doctor whether hormone replacement therapy should be considered

This leads to reductions in the efficiency with which calcium is absorbed from the intestine, and is followed by the compensatory PTH response described above. Consequently, the bone remodeling rate increases and bone is lost.

The response to these medications is actually more complicated, because they not only reduce vitamin D activation, but also directly impair the intestine's efficiency of calcium absorption. This is particularly true of the hydantoins. Such inhibition aggravates the drop in blood calcium, further increasing PTH secretion and bone remodeling. In addition, the hydantoin molecule itself exerts inhibitory effects on the osteoblasts in bone that replace the bone that has been removed, so that each remodeling event leads to an accelerated rate of bone loss.

Treatment of the anticonvulsant-associated bone disorder is generally successful and straightforward. Modest doses of extra vitamin D are generally sufficient to normalize the abnormalities in vitamin D concentration and calcium absorption. Some patients with particularly severe bone involvement may need higher doses and longer-term treatment to correct the changes observed on x-ray.

Bone health is an important concern for everyone, but especially for women. Women are more likely to develop osteoporosis than men because women have smaller body size and because they experience a sharp reduction in estrogen levels after menopause (testosterone and estrogen maintain bone density). Educational efforts to create greater awareness of bone health need to be increased (Table 16.1). It has been shown that institutionalized adults were protected from bone loss if they were given a daily supplement with vitamin D. Further, the economic impact of treating bone fractures far exceeds that of providing all patients with a small supplement of vitamin D. At doses of up to 2000 units/day, the risk of vitamin D overdose is very small. Therefore, it seems a reasonable public health strategy to provide all patients with a daily vitamin D supplement of about 400 units. Calcium intake should be 1500 mg/day for adolescent, pregnant, and postmenopausal women, and at least 1000 mg/day for reproductive-aged women. If dietary intake does not reach this goal, calcium supplementation should be considered.

For women over the age of 40 or those who are menopausal, bone density scans can be performed periodically to monitor bone health. This is especially recommended for women with a family history of osteoporosis.

Further research is needed into the effects of antiepileptic drugs and lifestyle on the bone health of women with epilepsy. In the meantime, regular weight-bearing exercise and good nutrition with special attention to calcium and vitamin D intake are recommended for every woman taking an antiepileptic medication.

SELECTED REFERENCES

Boglium G, Beghi E, Crespi V, et al. Anticonvulsant drugs and bone metabolism. *Acta Neurol Scand* 1986; 74:284–8.

Chung S, Ahn C. Effects of anti-epileptic drug therapy on bone mineral density in ambulatory epileptic children. *Brain Dev* 1994; 16:382–5.

Collins N, Maher J, Cole M, et al. A prospective study to evaluate the dose of vitamin D required to correct low 25-hydroxyvitamin D levels, calcium, and alkaline phosphatase in patients at risk of developing antiepileptic drug-induced osteomalacia. *Q J Med* 1991; 78:113–22.

Cummings SR, Nevitt MC, Browner WS, et al. Risk factors for hip fracture in white women. Study of Osteoporotic Fractures Research Group. *N Engl J Med* 1995; 332(12):767–73.

Gough H, Goggin T, Bissessar A, et al. A comparative study of the relative influence of different anticonvulsant drugs, UV exposure and diet on vitamin D and calcium metabolism in outpatients with epilepsy. *Q J Med* 1986; 230:569–77.

Sheth RD, Wesolowski CA, Jacob JC, et al. Effect of carbamazepine and valproate on bone mineral density. *J Pediatr* 1995; 127:256–62.

Stephen LJ, McLellan AR, Harrison JH, et al. Bone density and antiepileptic drugs: a case controlled study. *Seizure* 1999; 8(6):339–42.

Valimaki MJ, Tiihonen M, Laitinen K, et al. Bone mineral density measured by dual-energy X-ray absorptiometry and novel markers of bone formation and resorption in patients on anti-epileptic drugs. *J Bone Miner Res* 1994; 9:631–7.

Verrotti A, Freco R, Morgese G, et al. Increased bone turnover in epileptic patients treated with carbamazepine. *Ann Neurol* 2000; 47:385–8.

17

Psychiatric complications in epilepsy

Laura Marsh

Dr Laura Marsh is an Associate Professor of Psychiatry at Johns Hopkins University, where she is involved in research and clinical care. She has written a thorough chapter on the psychiatric symptoms that may arise in people with epilepsy. This is a problem that is often not recognized by health-care providers or by people with epilepsy. Yet, psychiatric symptoms are common. Up to 50% of people with epilepsy have depression, and depression is more common in women than in men. Anxiety, excessive mood swings, and irritability are other psychiatric symptoms that people with epilepsy may experience.

I had the good fortune to work closely with Dr Marsh when we were at Stanford University. She did important research there into how seizures cause emotional symptoms. She showed that people with epilepsy have *different* emotional symptoms depending on the area of the brain affected by the seizures. In addition to her work on the biological basis of emotional symptoms, Dr Marsh cared for many people with epilepsy. She knows first hand the difficult challenges epilepsy may bring.

In this chapter, Dr Marsh identifies environmental causes as well as biological triggers for psychiatric symptoms in people with epilepsy. She stresses that these symptoms should receive medical attention and discusses some of the safe and effective treatments that are available. After all, emotional health is an essential part of overall well-being.

MJM

Introduction

Almost everyone experiences emotions such as depression and anxiety. Often, people will 'explain away' feelings of depression or anxiety as understandable reactions to difficult circumstances. While this is sometimes the case, emotional experiences in women and men with epilepsy can also be a biological reaction to the epilepsy itself. In fact, doctors now recognize that epilepsy is associated with a number of emotional and behavioral symptoms.

Table 17.1. Psychiatric phenomena during the different phases of seizure activity

Ictal phase	Postictal phase	Interictal phase
Feelings of fear	Confusion	Adjustment disorders
Panic attacks	Depression	Major depression
Depressed mood	Agitation	Dysthymic disorders
Tearfulness	Aggression	Atypical depression
Sexual excitement	Paranoia	AED-induced conditions
Paranoia	Hallucinations	Psychotic syndromes
Hallucinations	Mania	Mania
Illusions		Panic disorder
Laughter		Generalized anxiety disorder
Forced thoughts resembling obsessions		Obsessive–compulsive disorder
Déjà vu and other memory experiences		Phobias
Confusion		
Aggression		

How often people with epilepsy experience psychiatric disturbances is not clear; reports tend to vary according to where the study was conducted. Studies based on patients from a community practice tend to show lower rates of psychiatric disturbance, whereas there is a higher rate among people with medically uncontrolled seizures seen at university-based epilepsy clinics. Nonetheless, epilepsy, like other conditions involving the brain, can be associated with psychiatric symptoms. These symptoms can have worse effects on well-being and functioning than the seizures themselves. In addition, psychiatric symptoms or illness can worsen epilepsy, as it is well recognized that emotional states can trigger epileptic seizures.

One of the most important aspects in the assessment of psychiatric symptoms in epilepsy is clarification of when symptoms occur in relation to the different phases of seizure activity; that is, whether the symptoms occur just before the seizure (the prodromal phase), during the seizure (the ictal phase), after the seizure (the postictal phase), or between seizures (the interictal phase) (Table 17.1). The cause of the psychiatric symptoms will be different depending upon whether they coincide with abnormal electrical activity during the seizure or are unrelated to seizures. Treatment approaches are also different.

Interictal depression

Mood disorders, particularly depressive illnesses, are common conditions. Studies suggest that up to 50% of people with epilepsy will experience a depression at some point. Doctors need to distinguish between normal feelings of depressed mood and psychiatric conditions that present with a depressed mood. The latter consist primarily of adjustment disorders with a depressed mood and depressive illnesses that have a biological basis, such as major depression, dysthymia, bipolar disorder (manic–depressive illness), subclasses of major depression with atypical features, and depressive disorders that are side effects of antiepileptic drugs (AEDs). Compared to adjustment disorders, the symptoms of depressive illnesses are more complex and affect physical, psychological, and social functioning more intensively. By definition, adjustment disorders develop after a stressful event. However, at least initially, depressive illnesses are frequently precipitated by stressful circumstances as well.

Feeling depressed for a few hours after a disappointment is usually a normal psychological reaction. Bereavement is also considered a normal psychological response, although prolonged symptoms require evaluation. Depressed feelings are regarded as psychiatric symptoms when they are persistently disruptive or cause changes in behavior that affect well-being and general functioning. The diagnosis of a psychiatric disorder is made when there is a combination of different symptoms and behavioral changes – not just a depressed mood. In general, interictal mood disorders in epilepsy have the same features as mood disorders in people without epilepsy. However, isolated psychiatric symptoms can also occur in epilepsy, such as in the context of seizures or as a side effect of anti-seizure medicines, and warrant psychiatric care.

Adjustment disorders

Adjustment disorders are diagnosed when a person reacts to a stressful circumstance or multiple stressors with significant changes in emotions, behavior, and functioning. The intensity of the distress and functional impairment is greater than would normally be expected in response to the stressor. Adjustment disorders with depressed mood are often accompanied by feelings of hopelessness or tearfulness, as well as suicidal feelings or suicide attempts. However, a wide range of symptoms can occur in adjustment disorders, including anxiety, irritable or impulsive behavior (such as fighting or reckless driving), or a combination of different emotional and behavioral changes. Adjustment disorders are not diagnosed if there is another more major psychiatric illness (such as major depression) that affects coping abilities and influences mood state. Sometimes, the symptoms of adjustment disorders persist and take on the qualities of a depressive illness.

Adjustment disorders typically develop within a few months after the stressor and then resolve. However, chronic or enduring stressors, such as chronic medical conditions or financial difficulties, may lead to persistent symptoms. Most people with epilepsy cope adequately with the experience of epilepsy, even though chronic recurrent seizures can be frustrating and disabling. For some people, however, the cumulative effects of seizures on relationships, employment, or daily functioning can become overwhelming and lead to distress. Many people find that distress and stress can provoke further seizures. For example, one patient who was having problems in a relationship had seizures whenever she spoke on the telephone to her boyfriend, but otherwise had only rare seizures. In addition, medication side effects, post-seizure symptoms, or memory problems and other types of cognitive (thinking) impairment further affect coping abilities.

Certain personality traits can make someone more likely to have an adjustment reaction. Therefore, it is best to consider individual circumstances and personality strengths and vulnerabilities rather than make sweeping generalizations about people with epilepsy as a group. For example, some people, regardless of whether they have epilepsy, have a greater emotional need to be taken care of by others; this may lead to too much dependency in relationships and to a greater sense of loss and disruption when relationships end. In people with epilepsy, however, dependency on others can also be a practical necessity because of recurrent seizures, rather than a personality trait. Whatever the case, emotional distress can result if relationships are disrupted and professional help may be needed to help resume functioning.

Major depression

Major depression is a common health problem that is very disabling, often recurrent, and tends to affect women more often than men. In the general population of the USA, nearly one out of every four women experiences at least one episode of major depression in her lifetime. Unfortunately, it can be difficult to recognize when someone has a major depressive episode, so many affected individuals are not diagnosed and never treated. This is partly because initial depressive episodes occur at times of increased psychological stress, and people tend to think their depressed moods are normal adjustment reactions.

The diagnosis of depressive illnesses always requires a professional evaluation. Women with epilepsy, however, should be alert to signs of possible depressive disorders. The main symptom of major depression is a persistently depressed mood or sadness, but loss of interest, self-confidence, or the ability to enjoy usual activities may predominate. Some people describe 'having no feelings' or 'not caring anymore.' Other symptoms of depressive illnesses are listed in Table 17.2. Usually, the symptoms develop slowly and worsen over time. Guilt feelings and a sense of worthlessness increase the tendency to find fault with oneself and to attribute problems to perceived personal inadequacies. Behavior is also affected. There may be agitation with pacing or hand-wringing, or movements may be relatively slowed, along with slowed speech and a tendency to sit around aimlessly and neglect usual tasks or work assignments. When symptoms are severe, personal hygiene may be impaired. These symptoms of depression cause profound problems in intimate and other social relationships, performance at work or school, and sexual functioning. With milder symptoms, activities require extra effort, but functioning may not be affected.

Suicidal feelings and suicidal attempts are among the most serious symptoms of depression. Studies find an increased rate of suicide in people with epilepsy when compared to the general population, underscoring the importance of seeking evaluation and treatment for depressive symptoms whenever they accompany epilepsy. Suicidal feelings in major depression may first start as feelings that life is not worth living. These may progress to recurrent thoughts of one's own death, or more specific ideas about suicide and how to carry out specific plans. Because depression makes people feel that they themselves are worthless, that things will never get better, and that there is no reason for hope, suicidal feelings often 'make sense' to the person who is feeling depressed. It is extremely important for people to realize, however, that these suicidal feelings will go away when the depression begins to subside. In this regard, treatment of major depression is often life-saving.

Table 17.2. Symptoms in major depression

Mood changes	Physical changes	Cognitive changes
Depressed or unhappy mood	Decreased sexual drive	Decreased ability to concentrate
Tearfulness	Decreased energy or feeling tired all the time	Decreased memory
Irritability or negativism	Insomnia or excessive sleep	Excessive indecisiveness
Decreased interest	Decreased appetite with weight loss (may also have weight gain with larger appetite)	
Inability to enjoy oneself	Increased physical complaints	
Withdrawal from previously enjoyed companions and activities	Excessive worries over health	
Decreased attention to oneself		
Neglect of duties		
Decreased self-esteem and self-confidence		
Inappropriate guilt or brooding		
Hopelessness, helplessness, or worthlessness		
Thoughts of death, suicidal thoughts or plans		

Dysthymic disorder

Dysthymic disorder is another common depressive illness that affects 3–5% of people in the general population. Some studies indicate that dysthymic disorder is the most common depressive condition seen in epilepsy patients. It is characterized by chronic symptoms of depression, which are present most of the time for at least 2 years. The features of dysthymic disorder are similar to those of major depression, but the symptoms are not as severe, and mostly consist of feeling somewhat sad or not being interested in usual activities. Feelings of pessimism, hopelessness, and helplessness are particularly common. Thus, dysthymic disorder can be very disabling, even though the symptoms are not as severe as with major depression. For example, in neurological disorders such as epilepsy, the presence of dysthymic disorder may lead a person to feel more disabled than is actually the case. Dysthymic disorder is also a significant risk factor for the development of major depression, a condition referred to as double depression.

Bipolar disorder

Bipolar disorder, also known as manic–depressive illness, is a mood disorder characterized by episodes of depressed mood similar to major depression, and episodes of mania or hypomania (a milder form of mania). In epilepsy, interictal bipolar disorder is relatively less common. However, some patients tend to have manic symptoms during the peri-ictal phase, often after a cluster of seizures.

An unusually happy or irritable mood is the hallmark of a manic episode. Behavior is affected because mania is associated with increased energy, optimism, and enthusiasm. This may lead to a decreased need for sleep, excessive talking, involvement in an unusual number of new projects, increased sexual interest, or risky, inappropriate, or even foolish behavior. People with mania often regard themselves as engaged in necessary activities and as very productive, although, in reality, behavior may be quite disorganized and nonproductive. Some patients with bipolar disorder will experience mixed states with features of both mania and depression. Also, there can be discrete brief episodes of depression during manic episodes. Patients with bipolar disorder are at risk for suicidal feelings or attempts during any stage of the illness. Therefore, proper treatment is crucial for maintaining function.

Atypical depressive syndromes

Some people with epilepsy experience atypical depressive syndromes or mood swings that are characterized by brief episodes of intensely depressed and irritable moods with periods of anxiety or an elevated mood, decreased energy, and difficulty sleeping. The periods of mood instability may last for only a few minutes, but their intensity can contribute to impulsive and distressing behavior, including suicide attempts. Further studies need to be conducted to determine how these syndromes are related to brain wave activity (as measured by an electroencephalogram), medication effects, effects of seizures on hormones, personality attributes, and features of bipolar disorder or major depressive syndromes.

Some women report disturbances in their mood during the premenstrual phase of their cycles, but whether these cyclical changes in mood are associated with variations in seizure frequency is unclear. At least one study has shown that women with menstrual-associated seizures (catamenial seizures) are more likely to have premenstrual tension than other women with epilepsy. It is important to note that many women who think they have a premenstrual mood disorder are actually suffering from a more persistent mood disorder, which may worsen during their premenstrual cycle. In other instances, women experience symptoms of premenstrual tension, characterized by irritability, depression, tension, anxiety, bloated feelings, a sense of weight gain, and changes in sleep and appetite patterns, but the symptoms do not significantly interfere with functioning. Therefore, it is important to monitor mood state throughout the menstrual cycle to establish the pattern of mood symptoms and whether they are related to other psychiatric diagnoses or specific personal issues.

Medication-induced mood disorders

AEDs commonly play a role in the development of mood symptoms. These effects are frequently dosage related, in which case lowering the total dose may relieve symptoms, although sometimes AEDs need to be changed. The use of more than one AED (polytherapy) also increases the risk of medication-induced mood symptoms. However, sometimes polytherapy is necessary to control seizures, and patients and their doctors must work together to arrive at a satisfactory treatment regimen.

The mood disorders brought on by AEDs can include depressive states that are remarkably similar to major depressive episodes. Others describe unexplainable irritability or mood lability, that is, unpredictable shifts in moods from tearfulness to joyfulness. Whereas some patients note immediate changes in mood after starting a new AED, others find that mood changes caused by AEDs occur more gradually. In either case, mood difficulties may be attributed to personal circumstances or uncontrolled seizures, underscoring the need for comprehensive psychiatric assessment when mood symptoms develop. AEDs can also cause sedation or negatively affect intellectual functioning, which further compromises coping strategies and mood stability. The effects of AEDS on brain hormones can also influence behavior.

Certain AEDs are more likely to affect mood and dull intellectual functioning, although virtually all AEDs are known to cause psychiatric symptoms. AEDs containing barbiturates (e.g., phenobarbital and primidone) and phenytoin are most often implicated, and carbamazepine and valproate are generally better tolerated. The newer AEDs gabapentin and lamotrigine do not appear to have negative mood effects. Felbamate is reported to cause extreme agitation, anxiety, or mania in some patients, and vigabatrin is associated with an increased frequency of psychotic symptoms. Benzodiazepines (e.g., Valium, Ativan, Klonopin) are useful for the short-term treatment of seizure activity. However, physiological dependence results from long-term benzodiazepine use, with the risk of withdrawal symptoms including severe anxiety or seizures when a dose is missed or the dose is reduced. Benzodiazepines can also make people disinhibited, sometimes leading to aggression or inappropriate behaviors. Brain damage and intellectual impairment increase the risk of benzodiazepine-related behavior problems.

Other interictal psychiatric disorders

Anxiety disorders

In the general population, anxiety disorders are the most common psychiatric illnesses among both men and women. Twenty-five percent to 44% of people will experience an anxiety disorder, with women affected two to three times more often than men. Typically, anxiety disorders are chronic, with symptoms generally starting in young adulthood. Often, anxiety and anxiety disorders are a prominent feature of other psychiatric conditions, especially depressive illnesses.

Up to one-third of people with epilepsy experience episodes of significant anxiety. Anxiety and stress frequently precipitate seizures. Symptoms of anxiety disorders also occur during seizures, and need to be distinguished from interictal anxiety symptoms.

As with depressed moods, doctors must distinguish between pathological anxiety and normal anxiety, as occurs with psychological conflicts, changes in life circumstances, or life-threatening or dangerous situations. Many people with epilepsy have fears and anxiety about having seizures, but they do not have anxiety disorders. Anxiety disorders refer to abnormal (pathological) states in which the intensity and duration of anxious feelings exceed what would typically be expected for a given situation. The evaluation of anxiety symptoms must also take into account that a number of medical conditions, including seizures, thyroid hormone disease, hypoglycemia (low blood sugar), and medications can cause symptoms that resemble primary anxiety disorders. Anxiety, normal or pathological, is characterized by uncomfortable feelings of apprehension and, often, a variety of physical sensations, such as sweating, chest tightness, stomach discomfort, headache, heart racing, or feelings of restlessness. Anxiety also affects intellectual functioning by interfering with concentration, learning, and memory. These physical symptoms of anxiety, in addition to advances in our knowledge of brain functioning, indicate that the experience of anxiety has a biological basis.

The anxiety disorders include generalized anxiety disorder, panic disorder with and without agoraphobia, post-traumatic stress disorder, social phobia and specific phobias, and obsessive–compulsive disorder. The main symptom of generalized anxiety disorder is excessive worrying or anxiety about a number of different issues, including minor matters. The anxiety is present most of the time, is difficult to control, impairs functioning, and is often accompanied by physical symptoms such as sleep problems, gastrointestinal problems, restlessness or edginess, muscle tension, headaches, and fatigue. Panic disorder, which affects about 1% of the population, is characterized by recurrent panic attacks consisting of brief episodes (about 30 minutes) of intense anxiety or fear accompanied by physical symptoms such as heart racing or shortness of breath. The panic attacks often occur 'out of the blue,' although specific situations may trigger attacks. Seizures can sometimes present with symptoms similar to panic attacks. Other signs of seizure activity should help distinguish interictal panic attacks from seizures.

Phobias are the most common mental disorders in the USA, affecting 5–10% of the population, and consist of irrational fears leading to the avoidance of specific objects, situations, or activities. Panic disorder can be accompanied by agoraphobia, which is the fear of being in public places. Agoraphobia can be severely disabling when it interferes with working or daily functioning. Social phobia, or social anxiety disorder, is characterized by disabling anxiety symptoms involving fears of embarrassment or humiliation in different social settings, such as speaking in public, at a meeting, or to a new person. Some people with epilepsy develop severe anxiety and fearful feelings about their seizures or about having a seizure in public. These feelings may develop into social phobia or agoraphobia. Such pathological anxiety states may actually precipitate seizures, and thereby reinforce the concerns about having more seizures.

Obsessive–compulsive disorder is estimated to affect about 2–3% of the general population. The features of obsessive–compulsive disorder consist of recurrent, unwanted thoughts, impulses, or images (i.e., obsessions, such as fearing something terrible may happen), and repetitive behaviors that the person feels driven to carry out again and again, often in a ritualized manner, for irrational reasons (i.e., compulsions, such as going in and out of a door or excessive handwashing). Attempts to resist carrying out the obsessions or compulsions result in increased anxiety, which may fuel further seizures. Epileptic seizures may consist of 'forced thoughts,' which resemble obsessions in that the thoughts are repetitive and their content is unwanted or unpleasant. Usually, the presence of other features of epileptic seizures help to distinguish between obsessions and seizures.

Psychotic disorders

Psychotic symptoms are characterized by disturbances in mental functioning that result in distortions of reality, referred to as hallucinations and delusions. Hallucinations are experiences of seeing or hearing things that are not really there. Delusions are false ideas believed by the patient, but not by others in his or her culture, and which cannot be corrected by reason. Interictal episodes of mania or major depression can be accompanied by delusions or hallucinations, but the symptoms go away when the mood disorder is treated. During manic episodes, delusions and hallucinations correspond to the elevated mood, and often carry themes of greatness or special powers, but also paranoia. By contrast, delusions in major depression tend to reflect depressive themes, such as thinking that one is dying or is guilty of committing crimes that never really occurred. Hallucinations in depression are often negative or demeaning, such as a voice telling the person 'You're no good.' Some patients with epilepsy experience chronic interictal psychotic symptoms that resemble chronic schizophrenia in that they are not associated with episodic mood disturbances. Psychotic symptoms are very serious symptoms that can lead to self-neglect, irresponsible or dangerous behavior, including self-harm. They are not influenced by reason, and reinforce beliefs about oneself that are brought on by the psychiatric illness itself, and not by reality. The presence of such symptoms should prompt medical evaluation.

Ictal and peri-ictal psychiatric disturbances

Ictal disturbances

A rich array of mental and emotional experiences may occur throughout a seizure, especially during the aura of the seizure (when consciousness is retained). These subjective aspects of seizures, sometimes referred to as experiential, were first written about in the 1800s by early researchers in epilepsy. For example, Hughlings Jackson described the 'dreamy state' in temporal lobe partial seizures in which recollections of past experiences combine with other mental phenomena such as hallucinations and illusions. In general, ictal psychiatric phenomena, like other clinical features of seizures, tend to be brief and stereotyped (meaning that the same symptoms occur during every seizure). However, these ictal changes in mood or other psychiatric phenomena are not always recognized as related to seizure activity. In addition, these mental experiences during a seizure can be very intense, leading some patients to feel emotionally distressed even after the ictal event has ceased. Sometimes, people do not feel well for weeks after an intense emotional experience during a seizure. For some patients, there may be feelings of hopelessness or even thoughts of suicide, which should be brought to the immediate attention of the doctor.

The range of psychiatric phenomena that occur during seizures is quite broad. One of the most common symptoms is anxiety, including extreme feelings of terror or panic during the seizure, a phenomenon referred to as ictal fear. While some people are anxious when they realize a seizure is about to begin, fearful feelings can also be caused electrical brain activity during a seizure, especially if the seizure begins in the temporal lobe. Ictal depression or tearfulness or crying seizures can also occur. When not recognized as a sign of seizure activity, these can be regarded as a reaction to some other life circumstance or as a feature of a primary mood disorder such as major depression. This assumption can mistakenly lead patients to seek psychotherapy or antidepressant treatment, when actually anti-seizure treatment is needed. Ictal laughter (referred to as gelastic seizures) is not associated with happy feelings, but tends to occur during a time in the seizure when awareness is impaired. Unfortunately, emotions such as joy, euphoria, pleasant moods, religious feelings, or sexual excitement are less common than negative emotions.

Psychotic symptoms may also occur during a seizure. Olfactory and gustatory hallucinations (the perception of smells or tastes which are not actually present) are often associated with partial seizures. Visual or auditory hallucinations may also occur. These hallucinations may consist of poorly defined shapes or sounds, although more complex visual scenes or speech can occur. Paranoid thoughts can occur and may be very frightening, even when the person knows the thoughts are part of a seizure.

Peri-ictal disturbances

Postictal and prodromal (i.e., before a seizure) psychiatric disturbances are related to seizures but are not directly due to the seizure activity. Prodromal disturbances are often described as a progressive build-up of tension, apprehension, irritability, depression or mood swings before a seizure. The symptoms can last for a few minutes up to many days until the seizure 'clears the air' and relieves the symptoms. Sometimes, ictal prodromes are associated with severe agitation, extreme mood instability, and impulsive behavior, which can cause social difficulties in addition to the distress felt by the patient.

Postictal psychiatric disturbances take a number of forms. The symptoms can last from minutes to several weeks. Emotional changes include both depressed feelings and mania or hypomania. Rather than elevated mood, postictal mania tends to be characterized by irritability, paranoia, and agitation. Postictal psychoses, often with paranoid features, tend to begin 1–2 days after a flurry of seizures and may last several days to weeks. During postictal delirium, consciousness and attention are disturbed and there may be confusion with agitated behavior, crying, or yelling. Violent or combative behavior may also occur, although usually this is because, during the confusion of a seizure, the person reacts to being restrained.

Risk factors and possible mechanisms of psychiatric illness in epilepsy

The development of psychiatric symptoms in people with epilepsy appears to be associated with a number of biological, psychological, and social factors (Table 17.3). Frequently, more than one factor contributes to the psychiatric symptoms experienced at a particular time. Studies in animals with epilepsy and other studies involving people with epilepsy have provided important information about the causes of psychiatric symptoms.

Biological factors

The most commonly cited seizure-related factors associated with psychiatric illnesses in epilepsy are structural brain injury, intellectual impairment, and effects of antiepileptic medications. These factors are interrelated in their contribution to psychiatric dysfunction. Brain injury may occur with head injury or stroke, as well as with injury present from birth, such as birth trauma or developmental brain malformations. With more extensive structural brain damage, there is a greater chance of psychiatric dysfunction as well as of intellectual impairment. Intellectual impairment in epilepsy can be quite variable. There may be no impairment, selective disruptions in memory, language functions, or other specific processes, or generalized impairment, as with mental retardation. More extensive brain damage is often associated with worse seizure control, requiring higher doses of AEDs or more than one AED. In turn, adverse medication side effects may be greater if there is brain damage or intellectual impairment.

The type of epilepsy and the location of the seizure focus are other possible risk factors for developing psychiatric illness, although this topic is debated. Earlier reports suggested that psychiatric disturbance was more common in people with temporal lobe epilepsy as compared to other types of epilepsy. Others suggested that certain psychiatric illnesses were more likely when the seizure focus was on either the right or left side of the brain. However, these findings have not been replicated consistently. Some studies suggest that having more than one type of seizure, rather than the location of the seizure, increases the risk of psychiatric disturbances. The age at which epilepsy began and the duration of epilepsy are not clearly related to the development of psychiatric symptoms.

Table 17.3. Risk factors for psychiatric disturbances in epilepsy

Seizure-related factors	Biological factors	Psychosocial factors
Structural brain damage	Familial predisposition	Unemployment
Antiepileptic medications	Hormonal changes	Low socioeconomic status
Intellectual impairment	Thyroid dysfunction	Social stigma
Multiple seizure types	Cyclical changes in estrogen/progesterone	Social isolation
?Temporal lobe focus		Family response to epilepsy
Poor seizure control		
?Age at epilepsy onset		

In order to stop ongoing seizures, the brain releases chemicals (neurochemicals) that can cause emotional changes and psychiatric disturbances. In particular, seizure-related changes in monoamine neurotransmitters may predispose to mood disorders and psychotic symptoms. Furthermore, epilepsy, especially temporal lobe epilepsy, often disrupts function in the region of the brain known as the limbic system. The limbic system includes a group of interrelated brain structures that are involved in the modulation of emotions and social behavior. These limbic structures have very specific connections to other brain regions that are also important to normal emotional regulation and to the development of psychiatric symptoms. Thus, epilepsy-related alterations in brain chemistry, especially in the limbic system, may lead to a 'neurochemical imbalance' that influences emotional functioning and behavior.

The role of reproductive hormones in the expression of psychiatric disorders and of epilepsy is of special interest to women with epilepsy. This area has not been thoroughly explored, but some studies suggest that variations in estrogen and progesterone levels during the menstrual cycle parallel changes in the frequency and severity of seizures as well as psychiatric symptoms, especially mood symptoms. In experimental studies, the seizure-activating effects of estrogen and the seizure-inhibiting effects of progesterone are well documented. Accordingly, some women experience catamenial (perimenstrual) seizures, which correspond to higher estrogen levels compared to progesterone levels during the luteal phase (second half) of the menstrual cycle. The cyclical fluctuations in estrogen and progesterone change neurochemicals that affect mood. AEDs and seizures themselves change neurochemicals and hormones. Perimenstrual mood disorders seem to improve with anti-depressants that act on the serotonin neurochemical system, suggesting that serotonin regulation may be disrupted in some people with epilepsy.

Genetic or familial factors are important to the development of psychiatric disorders, but whether people with epilepsy are genetically predisposed to psychiatric illness is not known. Several studies report lower rates for mood disorders or psychosis in family members of people with epilepsy compared to people without epilepsy with the same psychiatric disturbances. These data suggest that psychiatric-related illness is primarily due to epilepsy-related factors, rather than to genetics. Genetics do factor into the equation, however, and a family history of mood disorder appears to increase the tendency to develop AED-related depression.

Psychiatric illness affects men and women differently. In the general population, women have twice the rate of depression of men and are more likely to develop anxiety disorders. How gender influences psychiatric illness in men and women with epilepsy is unclear. Men are affected with epilepsy slightly more than women, but the rates of psychiatric illness in men and women with epilepsy are not different. A few studies suggest that men with epilepsy are more likely to have psychiatric symptoms such as depression, with more frequent suicide attempts and behavioral problems.

Psychosocial factors

Having seizures colors and shapes a person's life experiences and relation-ships. A number of life stresses associated with epilepsy can cause or worsen psychiatric illnesses, especially depression. These include perceived stigma associated with epilepsy, school difficulties, trouble finding and keeping a job, financial stress, and challenges related to housing, transportation, and social relationships. The unpredictable nature of seizures causes some people to feel they have little control over their life, a view that sometimes leads to despair and depression. Poor control of epilepsy may further increase isolation from others. Whether epilepsy begins in childhood or adulthood, families become overprotective and all these factors can affect psychological and social development.

Treatment

The first step in treatment is to identify, limit and, if possible, eliminate the risk factors for psychiatric *illness*. Many people with epilepsy can benefit from stress reduction and stress management techniques, such as relaxation training. Education about epilepsy is a very important method for reducing anxiety in people with epilepsy and their families. When the psychiatric disturbance is directly related to the epilepsy, as in peri-ictal psychiatric disturbances, treatment should focus on better seizure control. Then, if psychiatric symptoms do not resolve, the symptoms should be treated following approaches used for primary mental disorders.

Psychiatric symptoms caused by antiepileptic drugs

Psychiatric symptoms caused by AEDs are treated by lowering the medication dose or changing to a different AED. Psychiatric medications may be used to treat psychiatric symptoms while undergoing changes in the AEDs, and sometimes their continued use is necessary. When there are no other options, the AED causing the symptoms may be continued, with psychiatric medications also being used.

Adjustment disorders

The treatment of adjustment disorders usually involves psychotherapy and monitoring for the development of more major psychiatric illness. In general, psychotherapy provides an opportunity to ventilate emotions and concerns, identify life stresses that are especially problematic, and identify personal strengths and vulnerabilities that influence how one responds to stress. Psychotherapeutic approaches (described briefly below) should be individualized to the specific situation and person, and treatment can be either short term or long term, depending on the issues that need to be addressed. Medications can be used to treat disabling agitation, insomnia, or anxiety.

Major depression

The treatment of major depression includes medications, psychotherapy, or a combination of both. Antidepressant treatment reduces the the symptoms of depression and the risk of future episodes. When not treated, an episode of major depression typically resolves on its own after about 6 months. However, at least one subsequent episode of major depression develops in most people, many develop recurrent episodes of depression, and up to one-third suffer from chronic depression or only partial resolution of symptoms.

Antidepressant medications

Antidepressant medications act on different brain chemical systems and are classified accordingly (Table 17.4). All are equally effective in treating depression. However, a particular individual may respond better to one antidepressant than to another, and there may be a familial predisposition to respond better to one particular antidepressant. Initially, doctors prescribe an antidepressant on the basis of side effects. For example, a sedating antidepressant will benefit a person who is having trouble falling asleep. Because antidepressants work by changing neurotransmitter function, their therapeutic benefits may not be recognized for up to 6 weeks. Before determining that an antidepressant is not helpful, it is important to remain on the medicine for an adequate amount of time at an adequate dose.

Antidepressants are usually well-tolerated and the benefits of relieving depression symptoms far outweigh most negative side effects. One concern for people with epilepsy is that some antidepressants may lower the seizure threshold and and possibly increase the chance of having a seizure. However, the experience of physicians indicates better control of seizures when depression is treated. In addition, mood disorders in people with epilepsy respond well to relatively low doses of antidepressant medications. Antiepileptic medications and antidepressant medications may interact with one another, so the physician must consider potential interactions when beginning a new medication or adjusting the dose of an already prescribed medication.

Severe cases of major depression may require treatment with electroconvulsive therapy (ECT), which electrically induces generalized seizures. Although ECT is one of the safest and most effective treatments for major depression, it is typically reserved for patients who have not responded to antidepressant medications. Even for people with epilepsy, ECT may be necessary for the treatment of mood disorders.

Table 17.4. Classes and names (generic names with brand names in parentheses) of commonly used psychiatric medications

Antidepressants	Mood stabilizers	Antipsychotics	Anxiolytics
Nortriptyline[a] (Pamelor)	Lithium (Eskalith)	Haloperidol (Haldol)	Diazepam[h] (Valium)
Amitriptyline (Elavil)	Clonazepam (Klonopin)	Perphanazine (Trilafon)	Lorazepam[h] (Ativan)
Desipramine[a] (Norpramin)	Carbamazepine (Tegretol)	Thioridazine (Mellaril)	Chlordiazepoxide[h] (Librium)
Imipramine[a] (Tofranil)	Lamotrigine (Lamictal)	Trifluoperazine (Stelazine)	Alprazolam[h] (Xanax)
Protriptyline[a] (Vivactil)	Valproate, divalproex sodium (Depakote)	Fluphenazine (Prolixin)	Clorazepate[h] (Tranxene)
Doxepin[a] (Sinequan)	Gabapentin (Neurontin)	Thiothixene (Navane)	Clonazepam[h] (Klonopin)
Clomipramine[a] (Anafranil)		Molindone (Moban)	Buspirone[i] (Buspar)
Venlafacine[b] (Effexor)		Risperidone (Risperdal)	Hydroxyzine[i] (Vistaril)
Fluoxetine[c] (Prozac)		Olanzapine (Zyprexa)	
Sertraline[c] (Zoloft)		Quetiapine (Seroquel)	
Paroxetine[c] (Paxil)		Clozapine (Clozaril)	
Fluvoxamine[c] (Luvox)			
Trazodone[d] (Desyrel)			
Nefazodone[d] (Serzone)			
Mirtazapine[d] (Remeron)			
Tranylcypromine[e] (Parnate)			
Phenelzine[e] (Nardil)			
Isocarboxazid[e] (Marplan)			
Bupropion[f] (Wellbutrin)			
Mirtazapine[g] (Remeron)			

[a]Triclyclic antidepressants and norepinephrine reuptake inhibitors.
[b]Serotonin and norepinephrine reuptake inhibitors (SNRIs).
[c]Serotonin-selective reuptake inhibitors (SSRIs).
[d]Serotonin antagonist reuptake inhibitors (SARIs).
[e]Monoamine oxidase inhibitors (MAOIs).
[f]Norepinephrine and dopamine reuptake inhibitors (NDRIs).
[g]Noradrenergic and specific serotonergic antidepressants (NaSSAs).
[h]Benzodiazepines.
[i]Nonbenzodiazepines.

Mood stabilizers

Mood stabilizers are used to treat bipolar disorder and conditions with mood instability. Some AEDs are used as mood stabilizers, so that both conditions can be treated simultaneously. Lithium, carbamazepine, and valproate are the first-line medications for treating bipolar disorder or for irritability, changeable moods, or impulsiveness. Lamotrigine and gabapentin are newer agents that are also used to treat mood disorders. How these medications affect mood and behavior in people with epilepsy is not established, and they may aggravate behavior or cause depressive symptoms in some patients. Depressive episodes in people with bipolar disorder require antidepressant treatment. Psychosis can be treated with neuroleptic medications, and agitation is controlled with benzodiazepines. Lithium can provoke seizures in some people, although it is generally tolerated in people with epilepsy.

Anxiety treatments

Anxiety treatments include the benzodiazepines, antidepressant medications, specialized anxiolytics such as buspirone (Buspar), and psychotherapeutic approaches. The benzodiazepines, which are also anticonvulsants, should be used only for the short-term treatment of anxiety because tolerance and dependence on the medication result in more anxiety symptoms and potentially more seizures. Behavioral therapies, relaxation methods, stress management, or biofeedback are frequently used to help alleviate anxiety conditions. Relaxation training may be especially helpful for people with epilepsy because it helps people to regain a sense of control over their personal circumstances and, in some cases, can reduce seizure frequency.

Psychotic symptoms

Psychotic symptoms require treatment with a class of medications called antipsychotics or neuroleptics. Antipsychotics are used as adjunctive treatments to antidepressants and mood stabilizers in psychotic mood disorders; they are the mainstay of treatment for the chronic interictal schizophrenia-like disturbances. In addition to antipsychotic medications, psychosocial rehabilitation programs and supportive psychotherapy are necessary to optimize function. The newer antipsychotics, risperidone and olanzapine, appear to reduce both psychotic and negative symptoms and are fairly well tolerated. Personal experience suggests that people with epilepsy develop the motor side effects of neuroleptics at relatively low doses.

Psychotherapy

Psychotherapy alone can be used to treat adjustment difficulties, mild cases of depression, and some anxiety disorders. Otherwise, psychotherapy is best used as an adjunct to the medication management of mood disorders and psychotic disturbances. Psychotherapy is practiced by psychiatrists (medical physicians with an MD), psychologists (clinicians with a PhD), social workers, or licensed family therapists. All psychotherapy treatments involve a relationship with a professional therapist who provides an opportunity to examine one's particular circumstances and feelings and to develop strategies to improve function. Epilepsy Support Groups are not a substitute for psychotherapy or psychiatric treatment, but they help to reduce isolation and enable people with epilepsy to share information about epilepsy or personal coping strategies. Similarly, friends and family cannot fulfill the role of a trained therapist, but it is extremely important for people with epilepsy to develop friendships, personal interests, and a social network to reduce the impact of epilepsy.

Supportive psychotherapy helps patients understand how psychiatric symptoms shape life experiences and feelings and provides guidance and reassurance. The aim of cognitive therapy is to identify and replace negative-thinking habits that reinforce depressed feelings. The treatment is short term and focuses only on the resolution of current problems. Mild to moderate cases of major depression can respond to cognitive therapy alone, although the most lasting treatments include a combination of medications and psychotherapy. Behavior therapies focus on changing negative behaviors that promote depression or other symptoms and maximizing positive behaviors. Behavior therapies are commonly used for anxiety disorders, especially phobias, sometimes in conjunction with relaxation strategies and medications. Cognitive–behavioral therapy (CBT) combines principles from cognitive and behavioral approaches. For example, CBT may help people to focus on their capabilities, rather than on their disabilities.

Interpersonal therapies attempt to reduce symptoms by examining current relationships with others and ways of coping with stress. Family therapy helps patients and their families understand and deal with the symptoms of the psychiatric illness and of epilepsy, and aim to identify patterns of interactions that may promote better functioning. Group therapies can assist with the identification and resolution of interpersonal difficulties in social situations. Insight-oriented psychotherapy focuses on how depressive symptoms and maladaptive personality features relate to unresolved conflicts. Psychoanalysis is a very specialized form of insight-oriented psychotherapy that involves the exploration of unconscious feelings and inner conflicts in adulthood that result from certain childhood experiences. There is little indication for either psychoanalysis or insight-oriented therapy in the treatment of depression or other major psychiatric illnesses because the depressive disorder itself colors insight and perceptions about personal experiences. However, once the depression is treated, patients may wish to address certain issues using these approaches.

Summary

It is important to be aware of the different types of psychiatric symptoms that can occur in people with epilepsy and to encourage those who think or know they have psychiatric disturbances to seek evaluation and treatment. Even though many women with epilepsy show remarkable acceptance and adaptation to the recurrent seizures and psychosocial stresses associated with it, psychiatric disturbances are a common and troubling complication of epilepsy. The relationship between psychiatric symptoms and the consequences of recurrent seizures, factors that predispose to epilepsy, and antiepileptic medications is complex and not completely understood. Nonetheless, comprehensive management of the woman with epilepsy takes into account the fact that epilepsy raises the potential for developing psychiatric complications. The health-care providers and the woman herself recognize the importance of identifying and treating psychiatric symptoms in order to alleviate suffering and promote self-satisfaction and personal growth. With proper treatment, psychiatric disturbances can substantially improve or even completely resolve. Acknowledging that psychiatric disturbances occur in epilepsy and that they are treatable is an important first step for improving the quality of life of women with epilepsy.

Acknowledgments

This work was supported by grants from the Epilepsy Foundation of America, the Theodore and Vada Stanley Foundation, and the National Institutes of Health (MH-53485). The author is grateful to Scott Spears, MS, for research assistance.

SELECTED REFERENCES

Altshuler L. Depression and epilepsy. In *Epilepsy and Behavior*, ed. O Devinsky, WH Theodore. Wiley-Liss, Inc., New York, 1991, pp. 47–65.

DePaulo JR Jr, Ablow KR. *How to Cope with Depression. A Complete Guide for You and Your Family*. Fawcett Crest, New York, 1989.

Engel J Jr, Bandler R, Griffith NC, Caldecott-Hazard S. Neurobiological evidence for epilepsy-induced interictal disturbances. In *Advances in Neurology*, Vol. 55, ed. D Smith, D Treiman, M Trimble. Raven Press, New York, 1991, pp. 97–111.

Marsh L, Casper RC. Gender differences in brain morphology and in psychiatric disorders. In *Women's Health: Hormones, Emotions, and Behavior*, ed. RC Casper. Cambridge University Press, Cambridge, 1997.

Mendez MF, Cummings JL, Benson DF. Depression in epilepsy. Significance and phenomenology. *Arch Neurol* 1986; 43:766–70.

Nickell PV, Uhde TW. Anxiety disorders and epilepsy. In *Epilepsy and Behavior*, ed. O Devinsky, WH Theodore. Wiley-Liss, Inc., New York, 1991, pp. 67–84.

Reynolds EH. Biological factors in psychological disorders associated with epilepsy. In *Epilepsy and Psychiatry*, ed. EH Reynolds, MR Trimble. Churchill Livingstone, Edinburgh, 1981, pp. 264–90.

Robertson MM. Depression in epilepsy. In *Women and Epilepsy*, ed. MR Trimble. John Wiley and Sons, Chichester, 1991, pp. 223–42.

Seidenberg M, Hermann BP, Noew A. Depression in temporal lobe epilepsy. In *Psychological Disturbances in Epilepsy*, ed. JC Sackellares, S Berent. Butterworth-Heinemann, Boston, 1996, pp. 143–57.

Part V

Family planning, pregnancy, and parenting

18

Family planning and contraceptive choice

Pamela M. Crawford

Many women assume that they will have the opportunity to decide whether, and when, to have a child. Modern forms of contraceptives provide safe and effective birth control. The most popular form of contraceptive is the birth control pill. Introduced in the 1960s, these hormone-containing products rapidly became one of the preferred forms of family planning. Initial concerns that the estrogen hormones in these pills increased the risk for blood clotting and stroke led to the development of pills that contained very low doses of hormones. These products may lessen the very small risk of side effects, and the dose of hormone is no more than is absolutely necessary to stop ovulation.

In the 1980s physicians began to notice that women with epilepsy taking antiepileptic drugs and using birth control pills had more unplanned pregnancies than expected. Only one out of 100 women using birth control pills become pregnant each year – most by forgetting to take the pill on one or several days. However, women with epilepsy taking antiepileptic drugs had six or more failures per year per 100 women. Physicians quickly realized that some antiepileptic drugs increased the breakdown of the hormones contained within the birth control pill. Women were subsequently counseled that birth control pills could not be used safely when taking particular antiepileptic drugs. Unfortunately, many physicians still do not know about this interaction.

In this chapter, Dr Pamela Crawford reviews this complex and important topic. She stresses that each woman must know whether her medical therapy can interfere with hormonal contraception. Dr Crawford is a neurologist and specialist in epilepsy working at the Special Centre for Epilepsy at York District Hospital, England. She has a special interest and expertise in this area and has written and lectured widely on issues of concern for women with epilepsy.

MJM

Introduction

It is very important for every heterosexual woman to think about contraception and family planning, even before becoming sexually active. Nowadays, many neurologists discuss the issue of contraception with women before starting a drug to treat epilepsy. There is a variety of contraceptive methods from which to choose. These fall into two main groups – hormonal and nonhormonal methods. Contraception works *only* when it is used. No single contraceptive is 100% effective. The most common reason for women experiencing an unplanned pregnancy is because the birth control method was not used correctly.

Epilepsy treatment and effects on birth control

Epilepsy and its treatment do not alter the effectiveness of any of the nonhormonal methods of birth control. These nonhormonal methods include the intrauterine contraceptive device (IUD), barrier methods (cervical cap, diaphragm, and condom/sheath), the rhythm method and other methods of 'natural' family planning with or without spermicides, and sterilization (either tubal ligation for the female or vasectomy for the male).

Hormonal methods involve taking the combined oral contraceptive pill, (which contains two hormones, an estrogen and a synthetic form of progesterone called a progestogen), or the progesterone-only pill ('mini' pill), (Fig. 18.1), or long-acting preparations such as medroxyprogesterone (Depo-Provera) injections or a depot hormonal implant (Norplant) (Fig. 18.2).

Many women with epilepsy may have been told that they cannot take the oral contraceptive pill. This is now known not to be true. The reason that this belief arose was because some of the older drugs used to treat epilepsy speed up the metabolism (the breakdown) of the hormones contained within oral contraceptive pills. This results occasionally in an unplanned pregnancy. If a woman is taking one of the older antiepileptic drugs (AEDs) such as phenobarbital, phenytoin, mysoline, carbamazepine, or topiramate, she can still take the combined oral contraceptive pill but will need a high dose of estrogen; even so, the failure rate may still be higher than normal (Table 18.1). It is best to start with an oral contraceptive pill with at least 50 μg of estrogen and, if breakthrough bleeding occurs, an even higher estrogen dose may be needed. General practitioners, family planning doctors, or gynecologists may be worried about prescribing a higher dose of the combined oral contraceptive pill. However, the estrogen and progesterone which make up the pill are broken down faster than in people who do not take AEDs, so women

Table 18.1. Antiepileptic drugs that do and do not interact with hormonal birth control methods

Antiepileptic drugs which may interfere with hormonal birth control	Antiepileptic drugs which do not interfere with hormonal birth control
Carbamazepine (Tegretol)	Felbamate (Felbatol)
Phenytoin (Dilantin)	Gabapentin (Neurontin)
Phenobarbital	Lamotrigine (Lamictal)
Mysoline (Primidone)	Valproate (Depakote/Depakene)
[a]Topiramate (Topamax)	Vigabatrin (Sabril)
Oxcarbazepine (Trileptal)	Levetiracetam (Keppra)
	Zonisamide (Zonegran)

[a]Interferes weakly.

with epilepsy are not at any greater risk of developing complications such as thrombosis of the veins of the legs.

If it is very important that a woman does not become pregnant and if she is taking one of the drugs that speed up the breakdown of the combined contraceptive pill, she should use an alternative method of contraception or discuss with her neurologist changing her AED to one that does not interact with the contraceptive pill. Taking drugs such as sodium valproate, lamotrigine, gabapentin or vigabatrin for epilepsy means that a woman can take a normal-dose oral contraceptive pill without loss of efficacy. These drugs do not affect the speed of destruction of the contraceptive pill.

There are some types of hormone contraception that do not involve taking a daily pill. Medroxyprogesterone (a type of progesterone hormone) can be given as an intramuscular injection once every 3 months. This is called Depo-Provera. The advantage of this contraceptive is that it frees women from having to think about birth control every day. (Of course, this type of contraceptive does not protect again sexually transmitted diseases, as a condom does.) The dose of medroxyprogesterone seems to be high enough to work even in women taking enzyme-inducing AEDs. However, there are no studies directly evaluating the effectiveness of Depo-Provera in women with epilepsy.

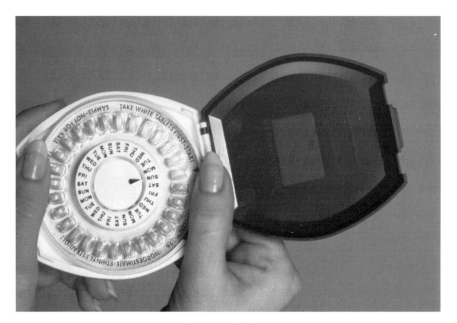

Figure 18.1 Progesterone-only oral contraceptive (mini-pill).

Norplant is a contraceptive system that utilizes a progesterone hormone (levonorgestrel) contained within small, silastic-covered rods. These rods are placed under the skin of the inside of the lower arm (Fig. 18.1). The progesterone is slowly released and the system protects agains pregnancy for as long as 3 years. However, Norplant has been associated with unplanned pregnancies in women taking AEDs that speed up contraceptive hormone destruction. It seems that the Norplant hormone is broken down so much by enzyme-inducing AEDs that it is not always effective.

Family planning

When a woman with epilepsy decides she wants to start a family, it is very important that she seeks help before becoming pregnant. It may be that she will not need treatment for her epilepsy during pregnancy or that she needs to change drugs or modify her medication dosage or schedule in order to avoid possible malformations in the developing baby. It is recommended that all

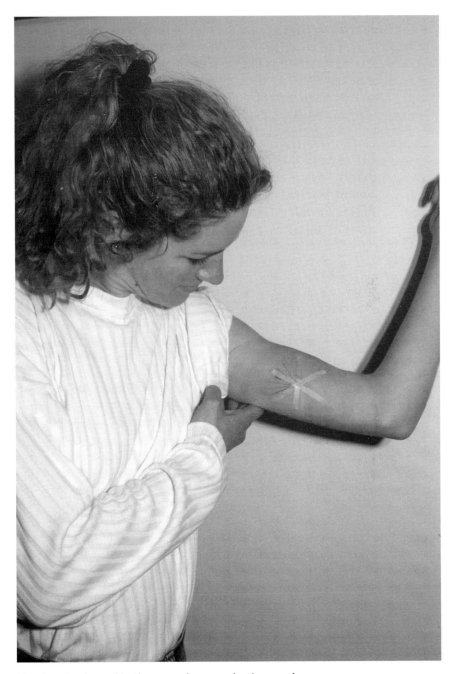

Figure 18.2 Norplant implanted in the arm of a reproductive-aged woman.

women start taking folate supplements for at least a month before conception. Because unplanned pregnancies can occur, many physicians recommend that all women capable of becoming pregnant routinely take 1–4 mg of folic acid each day. The advice that women are given today about pregnancy and contraception may be out of date in 5 years time. So it is very important that women regularly discuss their treatment and family planning with their neurologist, primary care provider, *and* obstetrician/gynecologist. It is especially wise to consult these doctors several months before becoming pregnant.

Nowadays, many neurologists discuss the issue of contraception with women before starting a drug to treat their epilepsy. However, do not wait for your doctor to bring the subject up – it is an important decision for every woman with epilepsy and usually requires some information and discussion.

19

Pregnancy risks for the woman with epilepsy

Mark Yerby and Yasser Y. El-Sayed

Making the decision to have a child can be joyous, as well as frightening. Every parent hopes that the pregnancy will be uncomplicated and the child will be born healthy. Women with epilepsy may be especially concerned that the risk of pregnancy complications and birth defects could be higher because of seizures and because the baby will be exposed to antiepileptic drugs. However, many women with epilepsy (and their physicians) believe these risks to be higher than they really are. Therefore, it is especially important for women with epilepsy to have access to comprehensive and accurate information in order to make an informed and appropriate choice. In addition, strategies to optimize seizure control, minimize medication exposure, and provide essential preconceptional vitamin supplementation need to be in place before pregnancy occurs. The information contained in the next two chapters should provide a good basis for discussion among women with epilepsy, their neurologists and obstetricians/gynecologists.

Dr Mark Yerby is a faculty member at the University of Oregon and an epilepsy expert who lectures widely on this topic. Dr El-Sayed, who provides the information contained in the boxes in Chapters 19 and 20, is an Assistant Professor in Obstetrics and Gynecology at Stanford University. He has special expertise in the gynecological and obstetrical care of women with epilepsy.

MJM

Reproductive health care is important for every woman. For a woman with epilepsy, regular appointments with her neurologist do not replace the essential visits to her obstetrician/gynecologist. Especially important is an understanding of how epilepsy affects a woman's reproductive health as well as of how her gynecological and obstetrical health affects her epilepsy.

Most women with epilepsy can become pregnant and have healthy children. However, their pregnancies are subject to a greater risk of complications, difficulties during labor, and a risk of adverse outcomes.

Box 19.1 General gynecologic health recommendations

The usual gynecological health recommendations also apply to women with epilepsy. All women should have a mammogram performed every 1–2 years between the ages of 40 and 49, and then annually. All women who are or have been sexually active or who have reached 18 years of age should undergo an annual Pap and pelvic examination. Following three or more consecutive satisfactory and normal annual Pap smears, the Pap test may be performed less frequently for low-risk women at the discretion of their physician. A digital rectal examination should accompany the pelvic exam and, after age 50, an annual fecal occult blood test should be performed. Sigmoidoscopy should be performed every 3–5 years after 50 years of age.

Yasser Y. El-Sayed

During pregnancy, one-quarter to one-third of women have more frequent seizures. Whether a woman will have more seizures appears to be unrelated to her seizure type, how long she has had epilepsy, or her seizure frequency in a previous pregnancy. Although an association was found between seizure frequency prior to pregnancy and increased seizures during parturition in one study, these observations have not been verified by other investigators.

A variety of hypotheses have been proposed to explain the increase in seizure frequency seen during pregnancy. Blood levels of antiepileptic drugs (AEDs) decline as pregnancy progresses, even if the AED dose is held constant or even increased. Yet, blood levels of AEDs tend to rise after delivery (postpartum). Whereas reduction of plasma drug concentration is not always accompanied by more frequent seizures, virtually all women with increased seizures in pregnancy have drug levels that are below the standard therapeutic range. There are several reasons why AED levels may drop during pregnancy, such as poor absorption from the gastrointestinal tract, a reduction in the blood proteins to which AED molecules attach, and increased clearance of the AED from the body because of liver metabolism and clearance by the kidneys. The rate of clearance appears to be greatest during the third trimester. Pregnancy-related weight gain may also cause drug levels to fall.

Sometimes, drug levels fall because of poor compliance with the recommended medication schedule. In one prospective study, it was found that more than one-third of pregnant women with epilepsy had more frequent seizures during pregnancy. Upon careful questioning, it was found that 68% of these women were not taking their medication as prescribed. In a Japanese study, seizures were more frequent in 27% of the women. One-half of these women were deliberately not taking as much medication as advised by their doctors because they were concerned about the effect the AEDs might have had on their children. To make certain that AED blood levels are kept within the most desirable range, many physicians recommend frequent monitoring of AED free levels.

It is important to maintain good seizure control during pregnancy, particularly the control of tonic–clonic seizures (grand mal seizures or convulsions). Seizures during the first trimester (the first 3 months of pregnancy) appear to increase the risk of congenital malformations. Generalized tonic–clonic seizures place both mother and fetus at risk for hypoxia and acidosis as well as for injury from blunt trauma. Canadian researchers have found that maternal seizures during gestation increase the risk of developmental delay. Although rare, stillbirths have occurred following a single generalized convulsion or series of seizures. Status epilepticus (i.e., prolonged seizures or a series of seizures lasting more than 30 minutes) carries a high risk for the mother and fetus. Fortunately, status epilepticus is an uncommon complication of pregnancies.

Complications of pregnancy

Women with epilepsy are at greater risk for other obstetric complications during pregnancy. Vaginal bleeding may be more likely to occur in women with epilepsy. Not surprisingly, anemia has been described twice as often in women with epilepsy as in those without it. Morning sickness (hyperemesis gravidarum) occurs more frequently in women with epilepsy, which may make it difficult to take oral medications. Also, pre-eclampsia has been described more frequently in these women.

Labor and delivery may give rise to more difficulties for women with epilepsy. Abruptio placentae (separation of the placenta from the wall of the uterus) and premature labor may be more common in these patients. Weak uterine contractions in women taking AEDs may require more assistance with delivery, such as induced labor, mechanical rupture of membranes, the use of

---

Box 19.2 Obstetric management of labor and delivery

Although the risks of such perinatal complications as poor fetal growth and intrauterine fetal death may be increased in patients with epilepsy, there is no clear consensus regarding what is appropriate fetal surveillance during pregnancy. Although the routine use of serial ultrasounds is controversial, any question on clinical examination regarding appropriate interval growth should prompt an ultrasound examination to detect a possible fetal growth abnormality or decreased amniotic fluid.

A safe and successful vaginal delivery can be accomplished in the majority of women with epilepsy. A tonic–clonic seizure is reported to occur in labor in 1–2% of women with epilepsy, and in another 1–2% of women up to 24 hours after delivery. Therefore, it is important to continue the administration of AEDs, especially during prolonged labor. Delayed absorption during labor can complicate the effectiveness of an orally administered AED. Intravenous or intramuscular administration may be necessary, especially in the setting of low serum levels or preseizure aura.

Yasser Y. El-Sayed

---

forceps or vacuum assistance, and cesarean sections, which are twice as common in women with epilepsy. Obstetricians caring for these women must be aware of the higher risks and be prepared to intervene.

Infant mortality

Fetal death (defined as fetal loss after more than 20 weeks of gestation) appears to be as common and perhaps as great a problem as congenital malformations and anomalies. Studies comparing stillbirth rates found higher rates in the infants of mothers with epilepsy (1.3–14%) compared to in the infants of mothers without epilepsy (1.2–8%). Some reports do not compare rates with general population figures or other controls, making it difficult to establish whether children are at increased risk. A large Norwegian study failed to demonstrate increased risks of stillbirth in the infants of mothers with epilepsy, but clearly demonstrated increased neonatal deaths.

Spontaneous abortions (defined as fetal loss occurring prior to 20 weeks of gestation) do not appear to occur more commonly in the infants of mother with epilepsy. A history of previous spontaneous abortions was not found to be significantly different between women with epilepsy (24%) and controls (17.8%). In one report, the gestational age-adjusted rate ratio for spontaneous abortions was no higher in women with epilepsy than in the wives of men with epilepsy. Nor was there any difference in spontaneous abortion rates for treated women with epilepsy (14.6%) compared to untreated women (15.7%). Other studies have, however, demonstrated increased rates of neonatal and perinatal death. Perinatal death rates range from 1.3%–7.8%, compared to 1–4% for controls.

Neonatal hemorrhage

A hemorrhagic phenomenon (i.e., related to bleeding) has been described in the infants of mothers with epilepsy. It differs from other hemorrhagic disorders in infancy in that the bleeding tends to occur internally during the first 24 hours of life. First described by Van Creveld (1957) and delineated as a syndrome by Mountain et al. (1970), it was initially associated with exposure to phenobarbital or primidone, but has subsequently also been described in children exposed to phenytoin, carbamazepine, diazepam, mephobarbital, amobarbital, and ethosuximide. Prevalence figures are as high as 30%, but appear to average 10%. Mortality is high (over 30%) because bleeding occurs within internal cavities and is often not noticed until the child is in shock.

The hemorrhage appears to be a result of a deficiency of vitamin K-dependent clotting factors II, VII, IX, and X. Maternal coagulation parameters are invariably normal. The fetus, however, will demonstrate diminished clotting factors. A prothrombin precursor, protein induced by vitamin K absence (PIVKA), has been discovered in the serum of mothers taking AEDs. Assays (blood tests) for PIVKA may permit prenatal identification of infants at risk for hemorrhage.

This phenomenon can be prevented by the maternal ingestion of oral vitamin K1 in the last month of gestation. AEDs can act like warfarin, and can inhibit vitamin K transport across the placenta. These effects can be overcome by large concentrations of the vitamin. Despite lower coagulation factor levels, the fetus is generally able to obtain enough maternal vitamin K *in utero*. After birth, the infant must rely on exogenous sources of vitamin K because the newborn gut is sterile. The routine administration of vitamin K at birth is not adequate to prevent hemorrhage if any two of the coagulation factors fall below 5% of normal values. Successful treatment requires fresh frozen plasma intravenously.

Low birth weight

Low birth weight (less than 2500 g) and prematurity have been described in the infants of epileptic mothers. The average rates range from 7% to 10% and from 4% to 11% respectively.

Feeding difficulties and drug withdrawal

Perinatal lethargy, irritability, and feeding difficulties have been attributed to intrauterine exposure to AEDs, especially to phenobarbital and phenytoin. Nursing children will often become sleepy and stop feeding prior to satiation. They will then awaken, hungry and irritable, to repeat the process. Some investigators have found no relationship between the type of AED, concentration, or disappearance from plasma, despite a twofold increase in sedation and drug-withdrawl symptoms in the infants of mothers with epilepsy. Virtually all AEDs are excreted in breast milk. The more highly protein bound the AED, the less will be transferred from plasma to milk. With the exception of carbamazepine and ethosuximide, the elimination half-life of AEDs (i.e., the time it takes for half the total amount of drug to be cleared from the body) tends to be prolonged in neonates.

Epilepsy in children of parents with epilepsy

The risk of epilepsy in the children of parents with epilepsy is higher than that in the general population. Interestingly, this risk is higher (relative risk of 3.2) for the children of mothers with epilepsy. Paternal epilepsy appears to have less impact on the development of seizures in children. The presence of maternal seizures during pregnancy, but not AED use, is associated with an increased risk of seizures in the offspring (relative risk 2.4). Evidence to support a genetic component for seizure development in these infants comes from kindling studies involving experimental animals. (Kindling studies are studies of one type of epilepsy in animals in which they develop partial onset seizures – temporal lobe seizures – after repeated daily electrical stimulation of the area.) If rats with experimental epilepsy are made to have generalized seizures during their pregnancy, their offspring are not more susceptible to kindling than rats with no seizures during parturition.

Management of the pregnant women with epilepsy

Those who care for women with epilepsy face a dilemma. On the one hand, seizures need to be prevented; on the other hand, fetal exposure to AEDs needs to be minimized. The ideal situation would be to withdraw the woman from AEDs prior to conception. However, for most women, this is not a realistic option. Women today are more likely to be employed and the potential disruption of their lives by seizures, such as the risk of the loss of their driver's license, makes the elimination of AEDs not a viable option.

Risk reduction needs to start prior to conception. Women (and their families) need to be educated about the potential risks before they become pregnant. Other risk factors for adverse pregnancy outcomes should be assessed and minimized, such as nutritional status (obese and underweight women have increased risks, vegetarians may not obtain enough vitamin B12), or other intercurrent illnesses (diabetes, phenylketonuria carriers, hypertension). There are other medications that are much more teratogenic (i.e., cause birth defects) than AEDs. Gold, lithium, iso-retinoin, folate antagonists, and warfarin are all teratogenic and should be avoided. Active maternal infections such as hepatitis B or a history of rubella exposure need to be established or ruled out. Measurements of the levels of antibodies to toxoplasmosis in the serum (toxoplasmosis titers) made prior to conception may help to determine whether elevated titers are secondary to a primary infection or an old exposure. Genetic risk factors such as Tay–Sachs, thalessemia, sickle cell disease, and cystic fibrosis should also be ruled out.

Risks can be minimized by the preconceptual use of multivitamins with folate and by using an AED in monotherapy with the lowest effective dose. Monitoring free drug levels (i.e., the amount of drug circulating in the bloodstream, unattached to protein and thus able to cross the blood–brain barrier and exert activity) both prior to and during pregnancy will permit accurate assessment of concentrations in a situation in which plasma protein binding is in flux. However, dose adjustment should be made on a clinical basis. Plasma AED concentrations will fall in pregnant women, but only one-third of them will have an increase in seizures. We tend to keep the dosage as low as possible during conception and the development of the organs, but will often raise it during the third trimester to reduce the risk of seizures during labor.

Supplementation with 0.4 mg/day of folate is recommended by the Centers for Disease Control for all women of childbearing age whether or not they have epilepsy. A number of observational and interventional studies have demonstrated a reduction in the risk of malformations in general and neural tube defects specifically in women taking folate prior to conception. The doses used ranged from 0.8 to 5.0 mg/day. All Western European and North American nations except Norway have similar 0.4 mg/day recommendations. The exception is for those women for whom there is a family history of neural tube defect. In these cases, 4.0 mg/day is the recommended dose. Ten milligrams of vitamin K1 per day should be initiated late in the third trimester to prevent neonatal hemorrhage. We usually prescribe it during the final month of gestation.

Seizures during labor and delivery are best managed with a parenteral benzodiazepine, although we have observed decreased fetal heart rates after intravenous lorazepam. During prolonged labor, a pregnant woman may not be able to continue taking her oral medications. Because medication withdrawl alone can precipitate seizures, loading with parenteral phenytoin may be necessary, especially for women with frequent generalized tonic–clonic attacks. Meperidine used as a post-cesarean section analgesic clearly exacerbated the myoclonic seizures of two of our patients. It lowers seizure threshold and should be used cautiously in patients with seizure disorders, including pregnant women.

Conclusion

A coordinated approach by both the primary treating physician and the specialist is important in promoting optimal treatment and adequate patient education. Despite the risks, with proper management, over 90% of women with epilepsy can have a successful pregnancy and healthy child.

SELECTED REFERENCES

Annegers JF, Baumgartner KB, Hauser WA, et al. Epilepsy, antiepileptic drugs and the risk of spontaneous abortion. *Epilepsia* 1988; 29(4):451–8.

Annegers JF, Elveback LR, Hauser WA, et al. Do anticonvulsants have a teratogenic effect? *Arch Neurol* 1974; 31:364–73.

Annegers JF, Hauser WA, Elveback LR, et al. Seizure disorders in offspring of parents with a history of seizures – maternal–paternal difference? *Epilepsia* 1976; 17(1):1–9.

Argent AC, Rothberg AD, Pienaar N. Precursor prothrombin status in the mother infant pairs following gestational anticonvulsant therapy. *Pediatr Pharmacol* 1984; 4:183–7.

Bardy AH. Seizure frequency in epileptic women during pregnancy and the puerperium: results of the prospective Helsinki Study. In *Epilepsy, Pregnancy, and the Child*, ed. D Janz, L Bossi, M Dam, H Heige, A Richens, D Schmidt. Raven Press, New York, 1982, pp. 27–31.

Bethnod M, Frederich A. Les enfants des antiepileptiques. *Pediatrie* 1975; 30:227–48.

Bjerkdal T, Bahna SL. The course and outcome of pregnancy in women with epilepsy. *Acta Obstet Gynecol Scand* 1973; 52:245–8.

Burnett CWF. A survey of the relation between epilepsy and pregnancy. *J Obstet Gynecol* 1946; 53:539–56.

Czeizel AE, Dudas I. Prevention of the first occurrence of neural tube defects by preconceptual vitamin supplements. *N Engl J Med* 1992; 327:1832–5.

Dam M, Christiansen J, Munck O, et al. Antiepileptic drugs: metabolism in pregnancy. *Clin Pharmacokinet* 1979; 4(1):53–62.

Dansky LV, Andermann E, Rosenblatt D, et al. Anticonvulsants, folate levels, and pregnancy outcome: a prospective study. *Ann Neurol* 1987; 21:176–82.

Davies VA, Argent AC, Staub H. Precursor prothrombin status in patients receiving anti-convulsant drugs. *Lancet* 1985; 1(8421):126–8.

Deblay MF, Vert P, Andre M, et al. Transplacental vitamin K prevents hemorrhagic disease of infants of epileptic mothers. *Lancet* 1982; 1:1247.

Eadie MJ, Lander CM, Tyrer JH. Plasma drug level monitoring in pregnancy. *Clin Pharmacokinet* 1977; 2(6):427–36.

Egenaes J. Outcome of pregnancy in women with epilepsy, Norway 1967–1978: complications during pregnancy and delivery. In *Epilepsy, Pregnancy, and the Child*, ed. D Janz, L Bossi, M Dam, H Heige, A Richens, D Schmidt. Raven Press, New York, 1982, pp. 81–5.

Higgins TA, Commerford JB. Epilepsy and pregnancy. *J Irish Med Assoc* 1974; 67(11): 317–20.

Hill RM, Tennyson L. Premature delivery, gestational age, complications of delivery, vital data at birth on newborn infants of epileptic mothers: Review of the literature. In *Epilepsy, Pregnancy, and the Child*, ed. D Janz, L Bossi, M Dam, et al. Raven Press, New York, 1982, pp. 167–73.

Holmes GL, Weber D. Effect of seizures during pregnancy on seizure susceptibility in offspring. *Epilepsia* 1985; 26:421–3.

Janz D. Antiepileptic drugs and pregnancy: altered utilization patterns and teratogenesis. *Epilepsia* 1982; 23(Suppl. 1):S53–S62.

Janz D, Fuchs V. Are antiepileptic drugs harmful when given during pregnancy? *Ger Med Mon* 1964; 9:20–2.

Kalen B. A register study of maternal epilepsy and delivery outcome with special reference to drug use. *Acta Neurol Scand* 1986; 73:253–9.

Kalter H, Warkany J. Congenital malformations. *N Engl J Med* 1983; 308:491–7.

Knight AH, Rhind EG. Epilepsy and pregnancy: a study of 153 pregnancies in 59 patients. *Epilepsia* 1975; 16:99–110.

Koch S, Gopfert-Geyer I, Hauser A, et al. Neonatal behavior disturbances in infants of epileptic women treated during pregnancy. In *Epidemiology, Early Detection and Therapy, and Environmental Factors*, ed. A Liss. Alan R. Liss Inc., New York, 1985, pp. 453–61.

Lawrence KM, James J, Miller MH, Tennant GB, Campbell H. Double-blind randomized controlled trial of folate treatment before conception to prevent recurrence of neural tube defects. *BMJ* 1981; 282:1509–11.

Leonard CH, Kilpatrick SJ, Schlueter MA, et al. Outcome of infants born at 24–26 weeks' gestation: II. Neurodevelopmental outcome. *Obstet Gynecol* 1997; 90:809–14.

Levy RH, Yerby MS. Effects of pregnancy on antiepileptic drug utilization. *Epilepsia* 1985; 26(Suppl. 1):525–57.

Lindhout D, Meinardi H, Meijer WA, Nau H. Antiepileptic drugs and teratogenesis in two consecutive cohorts: changes in prescription policy paralleled by changes in pattern of malformations. *Neurology* 1992; 42(Suppl. 5):94–110.

Monson RR, Rosenberg L, Hartz SC, et al. Anticonvulsants and parental epilepsy in the development of birth defects. *Lancet* 1976; 1(7954):272–5.

Montouris GD, Fenichel GM, McLain LW. The pregnant epileptic: a review and recommendations. *Arch Neurol* 1979; 36(10):601–3.

Mountain KR, Hirsch J, Gallus AS. Maternal coagulation defect due to anticonvulsant treatment in pregnancy. *Lancet* 1970; 1:265–8.

MRC Vitamin Study Group. Prevention of neural tube defects: results of the Medical Research Council Vitamin Study. *Lancet* 1991; 338:131–7.

Nakane Y, Oltuma T, Takahashi R, et al. Multi-institutional study on the teratogenicity and fetal toxicity of anticonvulsants: a report of a collaborative study group in Japan. *Epilepsia* 1980; 21:663–80.

Nau H, Kuhnz W, Egger HJ, et al. Anticonvulsants during pregnancy and lactation: transplacental, maternal and neonatal pharmacokinetics. *Clin Pharmacokinet* 1981; 7:508–43.

Nelson KB, Ellenberg JH. Maternal seizure disorder, outcome of pregnancy and neurological abnormalities in the children. *Neurology* 1982; 32:1247–54.

Otani K. Risk factors for the increased seizure frequency during pregnancy and the puerpurium. *Fol Psychiatr Neurol Japon* 1985; 39:33–44.

Ottman R, Annegers JF, Hauser WA, Kurland LT. Higher risk of seizures in offspring of mothers than fathers with epilepsy. *Am J Hum Genet* 1988; 43:357–64.

Perruca E, Crema A. Plasma protein binding of drugs in pregnancy. *Clin Pharmacokinet* 1981; 7:336–52.

Philbert A, Dam M. The epileptic mother and her child. *Epilepsia* 1982; 23:85–99.

Ramsay RE, Strauss RG, Wilder BJ, Willmore LJ. Status epilepticus in pregnancy: effect of phenytoin malabsorption on seizure control. *Neurology* 1978; 28:85–9.

Sabin M, Oxorn H. Epilepsy and pregnancy. *Obstet Gynecol* 1956; 7:175–99.

Schmidt D, Canger R, Avanzini G, et al. Change of seizure frequency in pregnant epileptic women. *J Neurol Neurosurg Psychiatry* 1983; 46:751–5.

Schmidt D, Nau H, Kock S, et al. Teratogenic and pharmacokinetic studies of primidone during pregnancy and in the offspring of epileptic women. *Acta Paediatr Scand* 1982; 71(2):301–11.

Smithells RW, Nevin NC, Seller MJ. Further experience of vitamin supplementation for prevention of neural tube defect recurrences. *Lancet* 1972; 2:839–43.

Speidel BD, Meadow SR. Maternal epilepsy and abnormalities of the fetus and the newborn. *Lancet* 1972; 2:839–43.

Srinivasan G, Seeler RA, Tiruvury A, et al. Maternal anticonvulsant therapy and hemorrhagic disease of the newborn. *Obstet Gynecol* 1982; 59:250–2.

Stumpf DA, Frost M. Seizures, anticonvulsants, and pregnancy. *Am J Dis Child* 1978; 132:746–8.

Suter C, Klingman WO. Seizure states and pregnancy. *Neurology* 1957; 7:105–18.

Svigos JM, Aust NZ. Epilepsy and pregnancy. *J Obstet Gynaecol* 1984; 24:182–5.

Tanganelli P, Regesta G. Epilepsy, pregnancy, and major birth anomalies: an Italian prospective, controlled study. *Neurology* 1992; 42(Suppl. 5):89–93.

Teramo K, Hiilesmaa VK, Bardy A, et al. Fetal heart rate during a maternal grand mal epileptic seizure. *J Perinat Med* 1979; 7:3–5.

Van Creveld S. Nouveaux aspects de la maladie hemorragique de nouveau ne. *Ned Tijdschr Geneeskd* 1957; 101:2109–12.

Vergel RG, Sanchez LR, Heredero BL, Rodriguez PL, Martinez AJ. Primary prevention of neural tube defects with folic acid supplementation: Cuban experience. *Prenat Diagn* 1990; 10(3):149–52.

Vert AP, Deblay MF. Infants of epileptic mothers. In *Intensive Care in the Newborn II*, ed. L Stern. Masson, New York, 1979, pp. 347–60.

Walker NP, Bardlow BA, Atkinson PM. A rapid chromogenic method for the determination of prothrombin precursor in the plasma. *Am J Clin Pathol* 1982; 78:777–80.

Yerby MS, Friel PN, McCormick KB, et al. Pharmacokinetics of anticonvulsants in pregnancy: alterations in plasma protein binding. *Epilepsy Res* 1990; 5:223–8.

Yerby MS, Friel PN, Miller DQ. Carbamazepine protein binding and disposition in pregnancy. *Ther Drug Monit* 1985; 7:269–73.

Yerby MS, Koepsell T, Daling J. Pregnancy complications and outcomes in a cohort of women with epilepsy. *Epilepsia* 1985; 26:631–5.

20

Risks of birth defects in children born to mothers with epilepsy

Aline T. Derdiarian and Yasser Y. El-Sayed

Dr Aline Derdiarian is a practicing neurologist and epilepsy specialist. She lectures widely on this topic. She is currently in private practice in California. This chapter also includes further information on gynecological and obstetrical care of women with epilepsy. This information should provide a good basis for discussion between the woman with epilepsy, her neurologist and obstetrician/gynecologist.

MJM

Introduction

Every pregnant woman wants to be certain that her baby is born healthy. Although women with epilepsy have a somewhat higher risk of having a child with a birth defect than do women without epilepsy, many overestimate the risk, partly because of the many misconceptions about epilepsy and pregnancy, even today. With the help of her physician or nurse, each woman with epilepsy can make a realistic assessment about the risks of pregnancy given her particular situation. It is important to remember that, with good preconception and prenatal care, more than 90% of women with epilepsy will have a normal, healthy infant.

Causes and mechanisms of birth defects/adverse outcomes

Birth defects include major congenital malformations and minor anomalies. Major malformations are significant physical defects which may be life threatening and generally require surgical treatment. Four to eight percent of children born to mothers with epilepsy have a major malformation, as compared to 2–4% of children born to mothers without epilepsy. Minor abnormalities are defined as variations from normal appearance that have no effect on health or well-being. It is more difficult to find accurate estimates of how often minor anomalies are found in children born to mothers with epilepsy. However, estimates are that 5–15% of children born to mothers with epilepsy have minor anomalies, which is twice the risk for children of mothers without epilepsy. Given the significant difference between the severity of major malformations and minor anomalies, it is important to distinguish between these two categories of birth defects.

The most common major malformation in children born to women with epilepsy is cleft lip and palate, which is a structural deformity of the roof of the mouth and lips because of improper fusing of midline bones and tissues. Other major defects include heart (cardiac) defects, which include ventral septal defect (an abnormal opening between the chambers of the heart), neural tube or spinal cord defects (including spina bifida), and urogenital defects (disorders of the urinary tract and genitalia). The risk that a child will be born with any of these major malformations is the same no matter which of the older antiepileptic drugs (AEDs) the mother uses during pregnancy. In other words, the chances of a baby being born with one of these birth defects are no different for mothers taking carbamazepine, phenobarbital, phenytoin, or valproate. The exception to this rule is neural tube defects, which are more common in children exposed to Depakote (valproate) or carbamazepine (Tegretol or Carbatrol) during the pregnancy. Approximately one to two out of 100 children exposed to Depakote, and one out of 100 children exposed to Tegretol will be born with a neural tube defect.

Major malformations are somewhat more common in children born to mothers with epilepsy – even if those mothers did not use AEDs during pregnancy. However, the risk is higher in women who take AEDs than in those women with epilepsy who do not take them. Therefore, we believe that AEDs are teratogenic, that is, that these drugs are capable of disrupting fetal development, causing birth defects. There is a great deal of interest in the scientific community about how these drugs might act as teratogens. An understanding of the mechanisms by which these medications cause human birth defects would allow medications to be developed that were free of these effects.

There are several ways in which AEDs can cause birth defects. Undoubtedly, more mechanism will be defined as clinical and scientific knowledge expands. All AEDs cross the placenta to enter into the fetal circulation. Some AEDs are metabolized (broken down) to free radicals (also known as arene oxides or epoxides). For example, Tegretol (carbamazepine) is metabolized to a 10, 11-epoxide metabolite. These unstable breakdown products may produce toxic effects by binding to other important cellular molecules. Enzymes called epoxide hydrolases or free radical-scavenging enzymes are responsible for eliminating these harmful metabolites. The level and activity of these enzymes vary in each individual and are determined by the genes. A genetic defect in these enzymes in one or both parents may increase the risk of birth defects in a fetus exposed to these metabolites.

Folic acid deficiency is another probable cause of birth defects in children exposed to AEDs *in utero* (as fetuses). Some AEDs cause a deficiency in the vitamin folic acid and others interfere with folic acid's biological activity. Folic acid is a vitamin necessary for the normal functioning of the immune system, nervous system, gastrointestinal tract, as well as the blood. A deficiency of folic acid has been associated with several major malformations – especially neural tube defects – as well as with minor anomalies.

Minor anomalies have also been reported in children exposed in utero to the older AEDs. It is not yet known whether the AEDs released after 1990 will have these effects. These minor anomalies can vary in severity from mildly recognizable to easily observed by trained physicians. Most of them involve the midface and fingers. There are no specific anomalies that are associated with use of a particular AED; rather, these types of abnormalities have been described with all of the older AEDs.

In the 1940s, trimethadione was a drug used to treat absence or petit mal seizures. Some children born to mothers who took this drug during pregnancy were short, had small heads (microcephaly), V-shaped eyebrows, prominent inner eyelid folds (epicanthal folds), low-set ears, irregular teeth, inguinal hernias, and underdeveloped penis (hypospadias). This drug is no longer available in the USA.

Subsequently, similar types of anomalies have been detected in children exposed to other AEDs. Dilantin (phenytoin) may cause small fingertips (distal digital hypoplasis), facial anomalies such as epicanthal folds, wide-spaced eyes (hypertelorism), a broad/flat nasal bridge, an upturned nasal tip, wide prominent lips, and intrauterine growth retardation. The syndrome associated with primidone includes features of upturned nose, long upper lip (elongated philtrum), straight/thin lips, small fingertips, low hairline, and lower birthweight. Phenobarbital use is associated with anomalies similar to those seen with phenytoin and alcohol exposure. Children exposed to valproate during pregnancy are reported to have epicanthal folds, flat nasal bridges, upturned nasal tips, long, thin overlapping fingers and toes, and abnormally shaped nails. Carbamazepine may cause epicanthal folds, abnormal eyelids, short nose, long upper lip, small fingertips, and small head.

In the last few years, several new AEDs have been introduced onto the US market, including felbamate (Felbatol), gabapentin (Neurontin), lamotrigine (Lamictal), topirimate (Topamax), tigabine, levetiracetam (Keppra), oxcarbazepine (Trileptal), and zonisamide (Zonegran). For the other newer drugs, it is still too early to know whether there is a risk of congenital malformations or minor anomalies, because there have not been a significant number of pregnant women with epilepsy exposed to these AEDs.

Preventative measures

With careful preconception and frequent prenatal evaluations, women with epilepsy can minimize their risks for birth defects and maximize their potential for good outcomes. It is very important that the diagnosis of epilepsy is accurate, that the most appropriate AED to control seizures is used, and that side effects are minimized. Whenever possible, a single AED at the lowest dose to achieve seizure control should be used. Major malformations are more likely to occur when mothers are taking more than one AED simultaneously, or receive large daily doses of medication. Risks can also be lowered if high peak serum doses are avoided throughout the day. This can be achieved by taking the same total daily dose but by dividing it into smaller doses taken more frequently during the day. Discontinuing or changing an AED that effectively controls seizures places a woman at risk for more frequent or severe seizures. Seizure control during pregnancy is important because uncontrolled seizures can injure the developing fetus or cause premature labor. Therefore, levels of the AED (the nonprotein-bound or free fraction) should be monitored routinely throughout the pregnancy.

Multivitamins with folic acid may reduce the risk of major malformations and minor anomalies. Folic supplementation appears to provide significant protection against neural tube defects. These vitamins are most effective when taken prior to conception. There are no clear guidelines on recommending the best size of dose of folic acid for women with epilepsy, but, generally,

1–2 mg of folate daily is adequate. If a history of neural tube defects exists in a prior pregnancy or in the woman's family, 4 mg/day is recommended.

Other preventative measures include routine and special laboratory studies, high-level ultrasound at 16–18 weeks' gestation and, if indicated, amniocentesis.

Box 20.1 Obstetric recommendations for prenatal diagnostic testing

At 18–22 weeks of gestation a comprehensive ultrasound examination to screen for congenital malformations (including cardiac anomalies) should be performed. The possibility of fetal neural tube defects (NTDs) should be evaluated with maternal serum alpha-fetoprotein (MSAFP) and ultrasonography, and amniocentesis offered for abnormal results. NTDs result from failure of the neural tube to close normally between the third and fourth week of embryologic development. The spectrum of NTDs includes anencephaly, encephalocele, and spina bifida.

The presence of an open fetal NTD will result in an elevated MSAFP level. MSAFP screening will detect approximately 85% of all open NTDs (80% of cases of open spina bifida and 90% of cases of anencephaly), with a false-positive rate of 3–4%. MSAFP screening will not detect skin-covered defects. Ideally, MSAFP screening for neural tube defects should be performed between 16 and 18 weeks' gestation, although it can be performed between 15 and 22 weeks. An elevated MSAFP ($>$2.0–2.5 multiples of the median) should prompt a comprehensive ultrasound examination to rule out fetal malformations.

Certain fetal intracranial ultrasonographic findings have been associated with NTDs. Ventriculomegaly, scalloping of the frontal bones, and downward displacement of the cerebellum have all been described. The sensitivity of ultrasound in NTD detection is probably greater than 90%; however, if an explanation for an elevated MSAFP cannot be determined by ultrasound, and if further evaluation is desired, an amniocentesis should be performed. An evaluation of both amniotic fluid AFP and the enzyme acetylcholinesterase is predicative of an open fatal NTD in greater than 99% of cases. Offering amniocentesis for amniotic fluid AFP and acetylcholinesterase to all women taking valproic acid or carbamazepine, regardless of MSAFP result, may be appropriate.

If an NTD is detected, extensive counseling should follow. Analysis of fetal chromosomes should be performed at the time of amniocentesis. The pregnancy management and neonatal prognosis should be reviewed, as well as the recurrence risks and prevention strategies. The patient should be given the opportunity to meet with physicians involved in the medical and surgical care of children with spina bifida, as well as with the families of children with spina bifida. The option of pregnancy termination should be addressed in nondirective counseling.

Delivery management is guided by attempts to optimize future neurologic function. The benefits of cesarean delivery remain unproven; however, the available data suggest greater retention of neurologic function in infants delivered by cesarean prior to labor. Cesarean delivery should be considered for women carrying a fetus affected with an NTD.

Yasser Y. El-Sayed

Conclusion

Most women with epilepsy have uneventful pregnancies and healthy, normal newborns. By understanding the types of birth defects seen in children of mothers with epilepsy, and some of the causes, a woman with epilepsy can take the appropriate steps to limit her risks and improve the health of her baby.

Box 20.2 AED Pregnancy Registry

The Antiepilepsy Drug (AED) Pregnancy Registry is the first North American registry for pregnant women who are taking antiepileptic drugs. The registry is maintained out of the Genetics and Teratology Unit of Massachusetts General Hospital in Boston. Women who enroll will be asked to provide information about the health status of their children. (All information will be kept confidential.) The findings will be analyzed to assess the fetal risk of antiepileptic drug use during pregnancy. The principal investigator for the registry is Lewis B. Holmes, MD.

Women and physicians are urged to call the registry directly at the toll-free number, 1-888-233-2334. For further information on the registry, please contact Massachusetts General Hospital – (617)726–1742 – or visit the website – www.massgeneral.org/aed

SELECTED REFERENCES

Morrell MJ. Pregnancy and epilepsy. In *The Epilepsies 2*, ed. RJ Porter, D Chadwick. Butterworth-Heinemann, Boston, 1997, pp. 313–32.

Morrell, MJ. Effects of epilepsy on women's reproductive health. *Epilepsia* 1998; 39(S8):S32–7.

Quality Standards Subcommittee of the American Academy of Neurology. Practice Parameter: management issues for women with epilepsy (summary statement). *Neurology* 1998; 51:944–8.

Seizure disorders in pregnancy. *Am Coll Obstet Gynecol Phys Educ Bull* 1996; 231:1–13.

Yerby MS, Leavitt A, Erickson DM, et al. Antiepileptics and the development of congenital anomalies. *Neurology* 1992; 42(S5):132–40.

Zahn CA, Morrell MJ, Collins SD, Labiner DM, Yerby MS. Management issues for women with epilepsy: a review of the literature. American Academy of Neurology Practice Guidelines. *Neurology* 1998; 51:949–56.

21

Neurocognitive outcome in children of mothers with epilepsy

Kimford J. Meador

Most women with epilepsy must continue taking antiepileptic drugs throughout pregnancy. The risk to mother and baby of seizures outweighs the small risk associated with exposure of the baby to antiepileptic drugs. Although health-care providers have some information about the risks of birth defects from exposure to antiepileptic drugs, we have far less information about the possible effect of these medications on the baby's and child's later intellectual and emotional development. In fact, there have been no good studies within the USA following children whose mothers took antiepileptic drugs while pregnant.

Dr Kimford Meador is a Professor of Neurology at Georgetown University Hospital and Chair, Department and an expert on the intellectual and emotional effects of antiepileptic drugs. He has recently received funding to perform a landmark study to follow babies whose mothers receive antiepileptic drugs while pregnant. The babies will be followed for years and the investigators will gather information on intellectual achievements, emotional functioning, and neurologic development.

In this chapter, Dr Meador reviews what we now know about the neurological and cognitive effects of antiepileptic drugs on the developing fetus.

MJM

The great majority of children born to mothers with epilepsy have normal intelligence. However, the children of mothers with epilepsy are at a slightly higher risk for a disturbance in the development of the nervous system that can cause lower intelligence, learning difficulties, and behavior problems. This is referred to as impaired neurodevelopment. The factors that affect neurodevelopment in the children of women with epilepsy are only partly understood. Nevertheless, reviewing what is currently known will help women with epilepsy make informed decisions and enhance their chance of having a happy, bright child. In addition, understanding the gaps in our knowledge will help women understand the importance of continued research in this area.

General factors affecting neurodevelopment

The combined effects and interactions of genes and the environment determine neurodevelopment. Thus, a child's neurodevelopment is affected by that child's inheritance, the mother's age at the time of pregnancy, the child's birth order, the mother's health during the pregnancy, drug exposure (medicinal and drugs of abuse), obstetric complications, the nutritional status of the mother and child, childhood illnesses, social and economic status of the family, the mother's and father's educational levels, as well as the child's educational opportunities. Inheritance accounts for 30–50% of the variability in intelligence (IQ). Although individual children can be severely affected by complications at the time of delivery or by severe childhood illnesses, in general, most obstetric complications and childhood illnesses do not affect the IQ. Malnutrition, to the degree that it arises in developed countries, does not appear to have a substantial impact on intelligence. Alcohol abuse during pregnancy can lower the child's IQ, but the effects of many other medicinal drugs are not known. Lower socioeconomic status may reduce educational opportunities in and out of the home environment. Further, children raised in poverty may not receive adequate medical care. Most scientists today believe that the chances that a child will have mental retardation are higher if the child has more than one risk. For example, approximately 50% of people with mental retardation have more than one of the risk factors listed above.

Human studies

Most investigations of neurodevelopment in the children of mothers with epilepsy find a slightly higher risk of developmental delay compared to children born to healthy mothers without epilepsy. Mental retardation is also more likely to occur in children born to mothers with epilepsy, but not in the children of fathers with epilepsy. Even though neurodevelopmental problems are more common in the children of mothers with epilepsy, the vast majority of children have normal intelligence, and individual children may have above-average intelligence. Multiple factors may combine to contribute to the increased risk of developmental delay in the children of mothers with epilepsy. Scientists have found that developmental delay in these children may be related to delayed fetal growth during pregnancy (intrauterine growth retardation), major birth defects, lower education levels of the parents, difficulties in bonding between mother and child, a partial seizure disorder in the mother, maternal seizures during pregnancy, and a higher dose or numbers of antiepileptic drugs (AEDs) taken during pregnancy. It is not clear whether exposure to AEDs during fetal development (*in utero*) affects intelligence. However, two recent human studies suggest that in-utero exposure to AEDs may cause behavioral deficits. In both studies, women without epilepsy in Denmark had been given phenobarbital during pregnancy for a variety of reasons. Years later, the adult sons from these pregnancies were tested and found to have lower than expected IQs.

Animal studies

Although there is very little information available concerning humans, animal studies suggest that there may be some negative developmental effects on the offspring of mothers taking AEDs during pregnancy. The negative effects may be more likely to occur in animals exposed to higher dosages and greater numbers of AEDs. Some mice exposed to phenobarbital *in utero* have shown changes in brain structure and brain chemicals, and behavioral disturbances. *In utero* exposure to phenytoin can cause impaired motor coordination and learning in rats. Similar, but less striking, neurobehavioral effects have also been seen in rats exposed *in utero* to trimethadione and Depakote (valproate). Dilantin (phenytoin) produces hyperexcitability and learning problems in monkeys following in-utero exposure. Animal studies of AED effects have the advantage of controlling for multiple factors such as the number of seizures, AED dosage and number of AEDs used, and heredity. It is important to bear in mind that findings in animals may not always be applicable to humans. Therefore, much more research in humans is needed to understand better the neurocognitive outcomes for the children of mothers with epilepsy.

Possible underlying mechanisms

A variety of factors may contribute to the neurodevelopmental deficits observed in the children of women with epilepsy. For example, seizures may interrupt blood flow and the supply of oxygen to the fetus. Seizures may also cause the mother to be injured and this could, in some cases, harm the developing fetus. Genes may also play a role. In some families, the genes for lower intelligence and for certain types of seizures may go together. People with seizure disorders may have more difficult social and economic challenges, which could negatively affect the development of their children. However, it is likely that AEDs are at least part of the problem.

Scientists have theories about how AEDs might interfere with brain development and with intellectual and behavioral development. AEDs may disrupt development by pathways similar to those that cause physical birth defects. The toxic metabolites (breakdown products) of AEDs are capable of attaching to RNA, DNA, or other proteins in the cells. These metabolites, called oxides or free radicals, could disrupt brain development. Individuals with inherited low levels of enzymes necessary to metabolize these toxic compounds could be at particular risk, because the levels of the toxic metabolites would be higher and the metabolites would be longer lasting. Folic acid is a vitamin essential for the synthesis of RNA and DNA – the building blocks of our genetic make-up. Several AEDs can reduce the level or activity of folic acid, and this might be one way that these drugs could interfere with brain development. AEDs could also disrupt neurodevelopment by reducing the activity of nerve cells (neurons) in the developing brain.

Conclusions and recommendations

Most children of mothers with epilepsy are developmentally normal. However, if there are any risks to the developing baby associated with the use of AEDs by the mother, those risks should be known so that physicians and women with epilepsy can take appropriate steps to minimize them. Such steps might include limiting the use of AEDs, maintaining excellent seizure control, and ensuring excellent nutrition and vitamin supplementation prior to conception and throughout the pregnancy. Most women with epilepsy do not have the option of discontinuing antiepileptic medication because the consequences of seizures can be more severe than any possible effects of AEDs. The present data suggest that AEDs can affect neurodevelopment, but the magnitude of these effects is uncertain. Further, the important question of whether there are differences between AEDs remains unanswered. Obviously, there is a critical need for further research to resolve these issues. Without such research, physicians will remain limited in the advice that they can offer, and women with epilepsy will not be able to make truly informed decisions.

Based on the presently available information, some limited recommendations can be made. Drug-induced birth defects and neurodevelopmental abnormalities occur primarily in the first few weeks of pregnancy. Because many pregnancies are not planned, every woman with epilepsy should discuss her particular situation with her physician, including whether treatment can be modified to reduce the risk to the fetus. Supplementation with folic acid should begin before pregnancy to ensure that vitamin stores are adequate at the time of conception. Treatment with a single AED as the lowest dose necessary to control seizures is recommended whenever possible. At this time, there is not enough information to know whether any one AED is better or worse than another. If a pregnancy is planned, a trial of AEDs might be considered if a woman has been seizure free for some years. However, this should be done only after consultation with her physician. For most women with epilepsy, continuing AED treatment is the best choice.

Children born to mothers with epilepsy have a slightly higher risk of neurodevelopmental difficulties, which can be reduced by good health practices, good seizure control, and using only as much antiepileptic medication as is necessary for seizure control. The vast majority of children born to women with epilepsy are completely normal. With more research, future outcomes will be even better.

SELECTED REFERENCES

Dansky LV, Finnell RH. Parental epilepsy, anticonvulsant drugs, and reproductive outcome: epidemiologic and experimental findings spanning three decades; 2: human studies. *Reproduct Toxicol Rev* 1991; 5:301–35.

Finnell RH, Dansky LV. Parental epilepsy, anticonvulsant drugs, and reproductive outcome: epidemiologic and experimental findings spanning three decades; 1: animal studies. *Reproduct Toxicol Rev* 1991; 5:281–99.

Fisher JE, Vorhees C. Developmental toxicity of antiepileptic drugs: relationship to postnatal dysfunction. *Pharmacol Res* 1992; 26(3):207–21.

Gaily E, Kantola-Sorsa E, Granström ML. Specific cognitive dysfunction in children with epileptic mothers. *Devel Med Child Neurol* 1990; 32:403–14.

Meador KJ. Cognitive effects of epilepsy and of antiepileptic medications. In *The Treatment of Epilepsy: Principles and Practice*, 2nd edn, ed. E Wyllie. Williams & Wilkins, New York, 1996, pp. 1121–30.

Reinisch JM, Sanders SA, Mortensen EL, Rubin DB. In utero exposure to phenobarbital and intelligence deficits in adult men. *JAMA* 1995; 274(19):1518–25.

22

Parenting for women with epilepsy

Mimi Callanan

Mimi Callanan is an Epilepsy Nurse Specialist at the Stanford Comprehensive Epilepsy Center. She has spent her career caring for people with epilepsy and is familiar with the concerns common to any new parents with epilepsy. In this chapter, she discusses the seizure-related risks of parenting a small child and offers reasonable and helpful suggestions to make a home environment that ensures your child's safety. I think you'll find this chapter reassuring. In my practice I have often met women with epilepsy who were told early in their lives that they should not have children because they would not be fit parents. Some women have carried that advice around inside themselves for years without ever challenging it. It is hoped that this chapter will make clear that being a parent is hard and wonderful for *everyone*. Women with epilepsy have special challenges that require some additional accommodation – but, after that, it's every Mom for herself!

MJM

The birth of a new baby can be one of the most exciting and fulfilling events in a woman's life, yet it is also a time of many fears and anxiety. The birth of a new baby requires major adjustments in life. These events may cause changes in roles and responsibilities within the family structure.

Planning a family for the woman with epilepsy cannot begin too soon. With the onset of menstruation or when her epilepsy is first diagnosed, the woman with epilepsy can work with her physician to discuss pregnancy and childbearing. Early planning can optimize the health of the woman during pregnancy and reduce the risks to the fetus.

Some women with epilepsy have fears of marriage and of having children. Well-meaning family and friends may try to dissuade them from having children for various reasons. These reasons may include concerns that the woman could not care for the baby if her seizures are not controlled, that pregnancy may exacerbate seizures, and that the baby may have birth defects, decreased intellect, or seizures. The choice to have children is an individual one and the decision should not be based on misinformation. Accurate information and counseling from professionals knowledgeable about epilepsy are every woman's right.

Once a woman with epilepsy decides to have children, there are a number of concerns that may arise. Fears common to all pregnant women include: the health of the children, their own health, parenting abilities, how they will deal with labor and delivery, and how they will manage child care. In addition, women with epilepsy are concerned that medications and seizures may harm the baby, that seizures may worsen during pregnancy, and that breastfeeding may or may not be a good option because the antiepileptic medication is present in breast milk. Many are concerned that labor and delivery will be complicated by seizures due to the stress of labor and because of the medications the obstetrician may give.

There are several special safety issues for pregnant women with epilepsy. Approximately 20–30% will have more frequent seizures during pregnancy; sometimes, this is due to sleep deprivation or because of missed doses of antiepileptic drugs (AEDs). Many women are afraid that AEDs will harm the fetus. Some women wonder whether it is better for their baby's health not to take medication. However, seizure control is important during pregnancy. Tonic–clonic and perhaps other types of seizures can increase the risk of miscarriage and of premature labor. Therefore, for most women with epilepsy, taking AEDs during pregnancy is the best decision. They should continue to take medications and have their blood levels of AEDs monitored. It is vital that pregnant women with epilepsy communicate often with their neurologist and obstetrician – both play a critical role in the woman's health and in the health of the fetus. Even if a woman's seizures are well controlled, it might be prudent to consider not driving during pregnancy, particularly if AED blood levels are fluctuating.

After the baby is born, new concerns about parenting arise. Bringing the baby home is accompanied by many feelings, ranging from excitement to sheer terror. In addition to these universal feelings, women may have concerns about sleep deprivation aggravating their seizures, and seizures compromising their child's safety. Depending on the woman, certain precautions may need to be taken in the home for the safety of the child, and adjustments in the woman's schedule may be necessary to ensure that she is well taken care of.

Precautions depend on the parent's seizure control and support. Sleep deprivation is a fact of life for all new parents. This can pose a major problem for the mother with epilepsy. Care must be taken to get plenty of rest. When the baby naps, it is easy to think of all the tasks that can be completed during this time, but every effort should be made to nap several times throughout the day with the baby. The baby sleeps less as it gets older and it becomes more difficult to catch up on lost sleep. If a woman breastfeeds, she can use a breast pump so that her partner can help with nighttime feedings, allowing her longer periods of uninterrupted sleep. If the baby is being bottle-fed, both parents can share the feeding responsibilities. In some instances, it may be advisable to ask family and friends to provide respite at night, or even during the day, so that the mother can get some sleep. Baby nurses (who stay overnight) are a wonderful option during those tough few first months of the baby's life for families who can afford them.

Medication adjustments may be necessary during this time. Doctors sometimes increase the dose of antiepileptic medication a woman is taking during the latter part of her pregnancy to ensure that the blood levels of medication remain suitably high, despite the faster breakdown and elimination of the medication during pregnancy. After delivery, metabolism slows and medication breakdown and elimination begin to return to prepregnancy rates. If a woman is breastfeeding, it may take longer to slow down. Healthcare professionals try to anticipate these changes, but some women may experience brief periods of medication toxicity if their metabolism slows faster than anticipated. On the other hand, if the medication dose is reduced too rapidly, seizures could break through. Women need to work with their physicians to achieve the right balance. It may be necessary to have frequent blood tests during this time.

Medication compliance is always difficult when a daily routine is disrupted. There is nothing that disrupts a daily routine more than bringing a newborn baby home. Day and night become almost indistinguishable during those first few weeks and a parent's schedule is entirely determined by the baby's need to eat, sleep, cry, be changed, and be held. It is easy to forget to take medicine or to become confused about the medication schedule. However, taking medication regularly and on schedule is even more important than during other times of life.

For the most part, women with epilepsy are no longer discouraged from marrying or having children. However, they and their health-care providers are still concerned that seizures could interfere with the mother's ability to provide care for her infant or young child. Some families may need to adjust their routines to provide safe parenting. When feeding a child, it is best to sit on the floor or in the middle of a bed with the back supported so that the baby is protected from falling if the mother should lose consciousness. A lovely room may have been designed for the baby, but it is safer to keep the baby next to the bed at night. Thus, when the baby wakes up, she or he can simply be lifted from the bassinet onto the bed. However, sleeping with a baby is usually not a good practice, even for the parent without epilepsy; pediatricians advise against it because a baby may be injured if an adult rolls over onto it. This risk of injury is even greater if the parent has a seizure.

When possible, family or friends should be involved in preparing bottles – one person can hold the baby and another can prepare the bottle. If a woman is alone, she should not carry the baby into the kitchen to make the bottle; it is better to leave it in the crib while preparing the bottle. When the baby is older, he or she should always be strapped into a high chair or infant seat for feedings. When it comes to changing a baby's diaper, the safest way to do this and to dress the baby is to sit on a pad on the floor (Fig. 22.1). If using a changing table, always strap the baby securely. Keeping diapers and infant care supplies on every level of the house limits stair climbing. Mothers whose seizures cause falls can place the baby in a stroller rather than a baby carrier, which could easily be dropped.

If bathing a baby in the tub, it is best for another person to be present, but, when alone, a sponge bath on the floor is perfectly all right. Also, when alone, a playpen or other enclosed area provides a safe place for the baby to play.

A child should never be held while cooking. Ironing or any other potentially dangerous activities should be delayed until another person is there. When a baby starts to walk, the house should be made as childproof as possible. Child safety experts suggest that adults get down on the floor and see how the world looks to a toddler. It is also important to think about what would happen if a seizure occurs and consciousness is lost. Outside doors should be kept locked and doors to rooms where the child could be hurt if not attended,

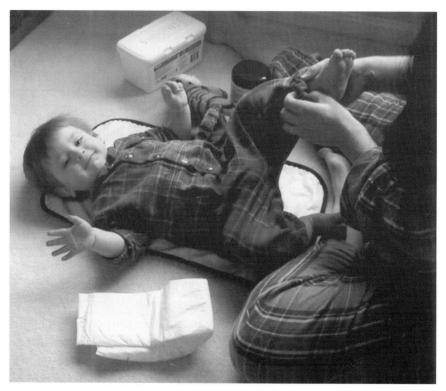

Figure 22.1 Changing a baby's diaper on the floor will help prevent falls in case of a seizure.

such as the kitchen and bathroom, should be closed. If a mother has seizures that make her confused or unaware, she should consider using a child safety harness or a wrist bungee cord to keep her child nearby when she is outside, and use safety gates at doorways and stairs to keep toddlers from wandering away. When it is time to toilet train, a child-size potty chair should be used rather than a booster seat on the toilet. Whenever a child is in the bathroom, the toilet seat must be down and cabinets and drawers locked.

Children should be educated about epilepsy and know how to respond if their mother has a seizure. Families can teach their toddler how to call a neighbor, relative, or friend for help if necessary. To help teach a toddler how to call for help, speed dial can be set up or the numbers on the telephone can be colored. A child who is a little older can be taught how to call 911 and how to give the home address. As the child grows, seizures can be explained in words he or she can understand. It is also important to use language that the child will not find frightening. Children may need to be reassured that they are not to blame for the seizures and that the parent will not die during a seizure. The mother's physician, the child's pediatrician or health-care provider, and a local Epilepsy Foundation can help in this process. It is important that the mother maintains her role as parent and does not let the child feel the burden of becoming the caregiver.

Parents with older children and teenagers may face different problems. Their children may withdraw from them and be embarrassed to be with them because the parent might have a seizure in public. Most older children simply need education about seizures to get over these feelings, although their parents will still generally embarrass them – after all, they are teenagers! If parent–child tension persists, family counseling should be considered.

One of the biggest fears women with epilepsy have is that their child will develop epilepsy (see Chapter 5). Although most types of epilepsy are not inherited, some are. When a child is diagnosed with epilepsy, most parents go through a grieving process for the loss of a 'normal' child. Reactions may include denial, anger, depression, guilt, and finally acceptance. Women with epilepsy may feel a strong sense of guilt. They may begin to remember all the warnings and advice from others regarding their decision to become mothers and question whether their decision to have children was right. The sense of guilt may be overwhelming to some. As she remembers her experiences with epilepsy, a mother may try to protect her child from all the bad experiences that she encountered as a child or young adult. Parental attitudes toward epilepsy affect the adaptation to it of both the parent and the child. If the mother has conflicting feelings about her epilepsy, her child may have a difficult time adjusting.

It is helpful to talk to other parents regarding common concerns and how they have handled them. Some of these concerns include: fears that seizures can cause brain damage or death; the effects of medication on intellect and long-term health; seizure first aid, both at home and school; and what to tell the school authorities. Other worries may include sibling jealousies and how to handle them; discipline and how to manage the fine line between being too lenient and too strict; the reactions of others, particularly other children, and teasing; how to tell others; how to deal with society's reaction; and finding good child care.

Parenting is one of the most exciting, fulfilling, and stressful experiences in one's life. Although women with epilepsy have special issues that need to be addressed and given thought prior to having children, they too can experience the many challenges and rewards of motherhood.

SELECTED REFERENCES

Devinsky O, Yerby M. Women with epilepsy. *Neurol Clin* 1994; 12:479–95.

Yerby M, Devinsky O. Epilepsy and pregnancy. Neurological complications of pregnancy. *Adv Neurol* 1994; 64:45–63.

Part VI

Living well with epilepsy

23

The impact of epilepsy on relationships

Patricia A. Gibson

For there is but one veritable problem – the problem of human relations. We forget that there is no hope or joy except in human relations.

ANTOINE DE SAINT EXUPERY
Wind, Sand and Stars

Patricia Gibson is at Wake Forest University School of Medicine in the Department of Neurology. She has provided information and referral services for people with epilepsy through the Epilepsy Information Service at Bowman Grey Epilepsy Center. She has also served as an advocate for people with epilepsy and has been deeply involved in educating nurses and social workers about epilepsy and the medical and social services helpful to people with epilepsy and their families. Early on, Ms Gibson recognized the special needs of women with epilepsy and organized one of the first national courses on this topic. In this chapter, she writes about how epilepsy may impact the important relationships in a woman's life – parents, partners, children, and friends. Ms Gibson offers practical advice to make certain that epilepsy remains something that a woman *has*, and never becomes something a woman *is*.

MJM

Epilepsy can have a significant medical, social, psychological, and financial impact. It can upset the equilibrium of the family system, affecting everyone in some way. Because epilepsy often begins in childhood, the patient's formative years may be drastically altered by the reactions of the family, school, and peer group to this disorder. A chronic illness of any type has significant impact on the lives of *all* the people it touches.

Epilepsy represents a varied group of neurological conditions, all of which include seizures. The social and psychological impacts of epilepsy are also varied. For some women, epilepsy is merely an inconvenience: a few seizures occur, medication is prescribed, their seizures come under control, and epilepsy does not interfere with life in any way. Most women with epilepsy are fortunate to be born into families who are knowledgeable and caring, to go to schools where the teachers are well informed and understanding, and to find employers who are enlightened, who judge them by their abilities and not by their epilepsy. Epilepsy is only a very small part of their self-identity and it becomes an ordinary part of life for this group.

Others may not be so lucky. For these women, epilepsy is a devastating diagnosis. Seizures may or may not be easily controlled. There may be other associated disabilities such as cerebral palsy, learning or behavioral problems. Their families may not be very knowledgeable about the disorder or the family unit may be struggling with other social and emotional problems. Their teachers may have little information about epilepsy and may be overprotective or rejecting. Uninformed employers and coworkers may engage in blatant discriminatory practices that make advancement difficult or even impossible for the woman with epilepsy. For this group, epilepsy is a major part of self-identity and daily life.

In my work with women with epilepsy and their families over the years, I have found that most go through stages in their adjustment to epilepsy. Many authors have written about these stages, stages that all of us go through in coping with any trauma. First, there is shock and disbelief ('How could this possibly be epilepsy?'). Almost always there is a stage of fear ('What might happen if I'm alone and have a seizure?'). Or, even worse, that nagging fear of 'what if?' ('What if others are there?'). The early stage of fear is often accompanied by bouts of 'bargaining' ('God, if you take this away, I will never smoke again'). This is frequently followed by stages of anger: anger toward God, parents, husband or companion, or even the health-care professionals. It is not uncommon for the affected person to experience feelings of guilt, as though she is somehow responsible for the disorder. She may feel guilty or inadequate when she is unable to control her seizures, when seizures appear to disrupt family events, or when driving or performing other tasks that contribute to family functioning becomes impossible. Many women, as they adjust to having seizures, go through a period of grieving and experience feelings of loss, often accompanied by depression. There is a 'loss of dreams' – a loss of perception that they are 'healthy' people with few limits.

Medicines have to be taken on a regular basis, driving privileges may be taken away, and career goals may have to be altered.

In time, most women come to an acceptance of their disorder and many develop philosophies helpful to their adjustment. However, not everyone goes through the stages as outlined. For example, one young woman who asked for epilepsy information a few years ago laughingly requested a packet of educational materials on epilepsy. 'I have an appointment with my neurologist this week', she said, 'and he is going to ask me again if I have called you to get information. You know, I think my doctor is more worried about this than I am. It's just epilepsy. My mother had it. It's no big deal. Send me something so I can tell him I have the information.' This young woman's recent diagnosis obviously had not been a major traumatic event for her.

Compare this to another young woman. When I visited her in hospital following the news of her diagnosis, she was devastated. Her mother was with her and had advised her daughter to tell no one about this awful news. Their social standing would be threatened in the community. Life would never be the same. Already, she was being taught to feel a deep sense of inferiority or inadequacy, that she was flawed and defective.

When epilepsy develops in early childhood, much of the adjustment depends on how the family adjusts to the disorder and helps the young girl cope with the ensuing issues and concerns (Goldin and Margolin, 1975). Certainly, the severity of the seizure condition, the presence of other handicapping conditions, the social, emotional, and financial stability of the family are all important variables. How disruptive the family perceives the disorder to be, regardless of whether their perception is accurate, is a key factor in their reaction. The family's adjustment to the diagnosis has a profound impact on how the child reacts. If the parents have a healthy attitude toward epilepsy and encourage normal functioning, the child can grow up with epilepsy in its proper place – just one part of what makes up that person.

This is especially important in relationships with siblings. When parents, out of fear and ignorance, focus constantly on the child with epilepsy, the relationships within the family become unbalanced and resentment and hostility build up. Often, it is the mother, as primary care provider, who becomes obsessed with watching the child constantly and fretting over what might happen. One mother became aware of her obsession when her daughter's drawings at school were displayed. In all the pictures where a mother was depicted, the mother had enormous eyes. 'I was shocked to find this image of myself', she said. 'I realized then that I was watching too much.' Another man, a physician, told of having a brother with epilepsy and other handicaps. 'My mom was "addicted" to my brother. She had no time for the rest of the children. Johnny's needs and desires always came first. We were all there just to serve Johnny. I am sure that is part of the reason I became a physician. Partly to help Johnny and thereby win my mother's love and attention.'

Many parents overprotect or overindulge the child with epilepsy, a practice that can be more disabling than the seizures. Parents who make the focus of their family life the provision of a quiet, pressure-free environment to prevent seizures make more difficult the usual interactions and development of normal relationships with siblings and peers. Young girls need these give-and-take interactions to role-play for later relationships.

Teenage years

The high-school years are a time of intense, and not always pleasant, emotions. As the young girl nears the teen years, her peer relationships take on much greater significance. The peer group becomes a new parent and may be more rigid and critical than the real parent. Physical appearance is crucial. 'Fitting in' is essential.

The teenage girl with epilepsy experiences a unique set of problems. The periodic, unpredictable loss of control threatens the autonomy that the adolescent is struggling to achieve. Susan Usisken, a young woman from London, once described her life with seizures as 'like walking on a series of trapdoors, any one of which may open and throw you to the ground without a moment's notice.' Certainly, living with this 'unpredictability' is one of the biggest challenges to those with epilepsy. During the teenage years there is also great pressure to conform in dress, talk, and thought. It is an age that allows few differences. Epilepsy can be mortifying, especially when the onset occurs during adolescence. Even if peers are accepting, the girl may feel stigmatized. This is the stage when relationships with the opposite sex are being explored. If the epilepsy is hidden, the young woman wrestles with the issue of when to reveal that she has it. Whom should she tell about the epilepsy and when? If she tells, does she risk rejection? Many young women struggle with this worry. This concern was taken care of for one young woman named Susan.

'No one knew I had epilepsy,' she told her support group one night. 'I was popular and running with the snobbiest kids in school. I was 14 and very "cool." I wore just the right clothes and had no time for anyone who was not just as "cool." Then it happened. I had a convulsion in the high school cafeteria during lunch time.' She paused for a moment and then revealed to the group, 'You know, that was one of the best things that ever happened to me. Oh, of course, I didn't think so at the time. My friends dropped me overnight and I was really devastated and depressed for some time. But then others whom I had never even spoken to wanted to know how I was doing. After a while I realized what true friendship means. I could have wasted my school years with those other superficial people whom I thought were my friends. I now view that seizure as a gift. It gave me an opportunity to learn who my real friends were.'

Another young woman who could not bring herself to talk about her epilepsy decided to put her medicine bottle out where her boyfriend could see it. When he picked it up and studied it, she held her breath. She wanted him to know, but just could not bear the thought of his rejection. 'Tegretol,' he mused. 'That's a medicine for epilepsy. Do you have *epilepsy*?" Her head fell and she barely whispered 'Yes.' He smiled and said, 'So does my mom!' And that was that. 'I just could not believe it. His mom! His mom has epilepsy!', she exclaimed. 'Since that day I shook loose of the hold that epilepsy had on me. And now when I mention having epilepsy, mostly everyone knows someone with it and they are usually eager to talk about it. I find that when I am open to and positive about it, so are most people in return.' Not everyone has such positive responses, and an early rejection sets the stage for social withdrawal and secrecy.

In the young and tender years when relationships are being 'tried on,' it is difficult to put these painful experiences into perspective. Not having that experience, the young woman depends heavily upon the opinions of peers to define herself. Certainly, being comfortable with herself *and* having epilepsy can be quite a challenge.

Denial of the epilepsy and rebellion against the limits that epilepsy imposes are not uncommon at this stage. It is during the teenage years that the restrictions of epilepsy are first and most keenly felt. If the seizures are uncontrolled, obtaining a driver's license, that 'American rite of passage,' is not possible. This can have devastating effects on the self-esteem of a young person and on her relationships. The car is an American status symbol. The ability to transport, especially in style, is a bargaining chip. The young woman who cannot get a driver's license has a downshift in her power. She becomes dependent on family and friends to go to the mall, to hold a job, to entertain.

Society's response to the young female's epilepsy affects and is affected by her personal adjustment. Those who have strong family support may actually make strides in altering the attitudes and behaviors of the less enlightened people in their community. Less assured patients will be greatly affected by the social slights, the cruel remarks, and the institutional prejudice they may encounter. The vulnerable ones may downgrade their ambitions, avoid competition, and be socially withdrawn. They become wary of society because it offers little security.

College years

Adult onset of seizures brings its own set of problems and concerns. Much of how this diagnosis affects the person and family will depend on their functioning prior to diagnosis and the family's understanding and support. In the college setting, the young woman may have to deal with her roommate's fears and concerns. Some patients report that roommates are frightened and ask to be moved immediately. Under the best of circumstances, learning to live amicably with another person in a very small space and under stressful situations is a challenge. Epilepsy only adds to that stress and poses strains on peer relationships during the college years. The young woman with epilepsy needs an environment in which she can get adequate sleep and rest, be free of alcohol and other drugs, and have a regular routine. This is certainly not descriptive of most college life, so problems may develop with close relationships during the college years. In earlier years, the parents would intervene to see that limits were set, but now the patient must take responsibility for her own care.

One young woman in counseling described her first year in college as the most painful learning experience in her life. Karen explained:

My parents had always controlled everything I did. They reminded me to take my medicine, told me when to go to bed, and constantly monitored my activities. We fought a lot during my last 2 years of high school. I resented their constant nagging and telling me what to do. I couldn't wait to get away and on my own. Looking back, I really wasn't pre-pared for the freedom of college. No one there cared whether or not I took my medicine. I had no limits on my time and I partied a lot that first year. It was wonderful until I had seizures and lost friends, especially after I lost my driver's license. My grades dropped and I was put on probation. It took me almost 2 years to figure out that I was now responsible for my own life and to recognize that I wasn't handling that responsibility well. It wasn't easy saying no to friends, I wanted to be popular, but I had to learn to care for myself first.

Karen found that, while there were lonely times during her attempt to regain control over her life, she also made new friends who supported her healthier habits. 'You have to learn to respect yourself,' she said. 'If you don't, then neither will others.'

Dating and establishing sexual relationships

One of the areas of great anxiety for both males and females with epilepsy is that of intimate relationships. The American culture worships physical perfection. These physical ideals have caused untold suffering and shame to many people. Indeed, it was only a few decades ago that laws were changed in the USA that allowed marriages to be annulled if one of the partners was found to have epilepsy. In India today, an annulment is expected should the woman be found to have epilepsy. The woman is looked upon as 'damaged goods,' which can and should be returned. Fortunately, efforts are underway to change these outmoded views of women, but this change does not occur quickly.

Women experience many fears concerning the formation of intimate and sexual relationships: the worry that sexual partners will not find them attractive, that they will be rejected once the epilepsy is revealed, or that they will have seizures during sex. Rejection does occur on occasion, as it does for many women who do not have epilepsy. A woman with epilepsy needs to be careful not to place too much emphasis on her condition. It is only a small part of who she is. People who run from relationships on the basis of learning about the epilepsy are not really ready for a mature relationship. I once sat beside a man on an overseas airplane trip who, after learning of my work, confided that he had been very attracted to a young woman in high school. On their first date, the young woman had a convulsive seizure. He was frightened, took her home, and never asked her out again. It was never discussed with anyone. 'That young woman is now a member of Parliament, well thought of by everyone,' he went on. 'She has accomplished so much. I was so young and silly. I missed out on getting to know an outstanding person because of my fears,' he said regretfully.

Not everyone experiences rejection; many women report extraordinary experiences when they confided that they had epilepsy to their boyfriends. 'When I told him I had epilepsy, he just looked at me with such love and said, "So?" It is the most wonderful feeling to be loved just as you are, epilepsy and all,' reported one woman from North Carolina.

One of the biggest steps for the woman with epilepsy is to build a good relationship with herself, to become self-accepting. Merle Shain, in her book *When Lovers Are Friends*, said:

We are all connected to the world by a thousand hidden strings that we don't see. There are the strings of other people's expectations and those we make ourselves out of vanity or fear. And the world is very quick to hang a myth on you which can cover you like a net, and if you aren't nimble enough to jump clear of it you can spend your life inside.

So it is true of epilepsy and the net that others may try to throw over the woman affected.

Poor self-esteem is rampant in woman today and especially so in women with any chronic health problem. When women lack self-esteem, they are more at risk of becoming involved in unhealthy relationships. In a survey conducted by Dr Paul Schraeder, of the 51 consecutive women with epilepsy referred to a university hospital epilepsy practice in New Jersey, 32% reported sexual abuse as children; 31% were physically abused as children; 34% reported physical abuse as adults by a partner. Over 50% of the women reported physical or sexual abuse in their lifetime, compared to the combined rate reported in a community-based primary health-care setting of 30%. In a recent survey of women with epilepsy by the author, a number of the women reported being sexually promiscuous in their early years due to their concern that no one would love them. Sex was a means to prove their attractiveness. One woman wrote:

I don't remember a lot of my past. I feel like the only things I remember are the bad things that happened to me. My seizures got worse when I was 8 and was molested by a preacher. Later, in high school, I never really dated and I only had a few friends. I had sex but I never liked it. I think I done it because I was looking for acceptance and for someone to love me the way I always wanted to be loved.

This young woman's early insight helped her to pursue counseling and she is now happily married, although continuing to struggle with uncontrolled seizures and poor self-esteem.

Marriage and parenthood

Marriage brings with it expectations of shared tasks. If seizures are uncontrolled, there may be strains on the marital relationship when the woman with epilepsy cannot fulfill her role as expected. In a recent unpublished study on quality of life assessment in women with epilepsy conducted by Shumacher and others, it was found that loss of a driver's license was of great concern. This was the second most frequently mentioned area in the list of negative aspects of living with epilepsy. The open-ended responses not only revealed the ways in which epilepsy can affect a woman on many levels, but also made clear the relationships between this legal restriction and a woman's personal, familial, social, and economic well-being. For these women, driving restrictions meant functional restrictions, the loss of independence, social isolation, increased economic burden, diminished personal safety and self-esteem, and loss of the intrinsic pleasure of driving. Grocery shopping, getting to medical appointments, and getting to and from work become daunting tasks. Having to be dependent on others was noted to be especially difficult. One woman with three young children compared her situation to 'being in prison.' Her family lives in an isolated area. Her whole life revolves around her husband's schedule and she has few friends. Her husband's family lives in the town nearby, but seems to resent any requests for lifts. She feels depressed much of the time.

The parental relationship with children can also be affected by epilepsy. Much of how the relationship develops depends on the children's early understanding of the epilepsy. When the seizures are surrounded by fears and misconceptions and no attempts are made to educate the children, relationships may be severely affected. If the seizures are uncontrolled, the oldest child often becomes the 'caretaker'. He or she may become obsessed with the mother's well-being and constantly check on this. Small children may fear abandonment by the parent. Considerable anxiety may be prevalent in the home. The children may worry that the parent is going to die or may that they, too, will develop seizures. Without reliable information, the children begin to form their own distorted perceptions about what is taking place. Some parents, not wanting to burden their children, may try to keep the epilepsy secret. When the child learns that this condition has existed for years, he or she may become distrustful. Without healthy discussion of the facts, the child has to depend upon other sources for information, such as friends, television, books, and the Internet, which may or may not be accurate.

Some years ago, Lechtenberg and Akner conducted a study of children who had a parent with epilepsy. They looked at the impact of this disorder on the children and their adjustment and coping skills. They found that young children allowed to see the parent's seizures and the treatment for those seizures adapted to the threat of illness in a parent by becoming involved in his or her care and supervision. Parents who concealed their disorder actually faced the most anger and resentment from their children. The authors maintained that a clear explanation and disclosure of the problem to the children, regardless of their ages, was the best approach to maintaining healthy relationships with the parents.

When the mother's seizures are uncontrolled, the caretaking role may be usurped by others, often the grandmother. I counseled one woman whose husband left her and her two daughters. Because of the frequency and severity of her seizures, she found it necessary to move in with her parents. In time the grandmother took over more and more of the parenting role with the daughters. The patient admitted:

There were times, because of the seizures and the heavy medication, that I was unable to attend to their needs. However, as I got better I found myself being pushed back and treated more like one of the young children. This dismissal of myself as a parent was damaging to my relationship with my children. It was a very difficult time in my life. I truly appreciated the help of my mother, but she went beyond helping to completely taking over my role as a parent. I also think her response to my seizures was exaggerated. This worsened the children's fears, thus increasing their dependency on her. It was very difficult to build up the self-confidence to confront her about this. I realized I had to move out if I were to establish a normal parenting relationship with my children.

It has long been of great interest to me to observe how some women cope so well with epilepsy while others struggle. How a particular predicament is experienced depends largely upon the individual's character, as well as on the severity of her seizures and her response to treatment. For each person, the experience with epilepsy will be a little different, but the following are some suggestions of coping strategies.

1 The woman with epilepsy should get as much information as possible about the disorder. She must become the 'expert' on it. No doctor or other professional is going to be as interested in her care as she is. She must know the names of her medicines, the doses; and seizure type, keep a seizure calendar, keep track of the times of her seizure, what she was doing at the time, and look for any patterns that develop.

2 The woman must become a partner with her doctor in the treatment. She should be willing to look at her own actions that may be causing problems and see what can be changed to improve her condition. I have talked with many women who complained of having seizures and later in our conversation acknowledged they had missed their medication or were not taking it as prescribed or were drinking alcohol, going without sleep, etc. Yet they saw their uncontrolled seizures as the doctor's responsibility.

3 The woman with epilepsy should be informed enough to teach others about epilepsy, and to teach it well and in a positive manner. This often makes a difference to how others react to her. Most people will welcome an opportunity to learn about the condition.

4 When first diagnosed, epilepsy may be chief among a woman's concerns. At some point, however, she needs to let it go and not allow it to become the focus of her life. After time, it should not be the main topic of conversation with family or friends. It is important to get on with life. This is not easy when seizures are uncontrolled and frequent, but even then it is not necessary to let the seizures take over all conversations and be the main focus of life.

5 If she continues to worry excessively and is having difficulties with relationships, the woman with epilepsy should seek counseling. It is very helpful to have someone outside the family with whom to voice fears, worries, and concerns. A doctor or people in local epilepsy groups can offer recommendations about this.

6 It is important to develop a social network. One of the best ways to feel good about oneself is to form relationships with others who accept the whole person and respond positively. This requires some risk taking and time to find the right group of people.

There is no way to learn without making errors. I know of no one who has not made errors in establishing relationships. Mistakes are information about what works and what does not work. They have nothing to do with self-worth; they are merely steps to a better relationship.

Establishing and maintaining relationships are not easy for anyone. According to Merle Shain, 'there are only two ways to approach life – as victim or as gallant fighter – and you must decide if you want to act or react, deal your own cards or play with a stacked deck. And if you don't decide which way to play with life, it always plays with you.' In *A Farewell to Arms*, Ernest Hemingway writes: 'The world breaks everyone and afterward many are strong at the broken places.' Although epilepsy does not 'break' a person, living with epilepsy can pose many challenges. However, with the support of family, friends, and health-care providers, women can realize that although epilepsy affects their lives, it does not define their lives.

SELECTED REFERENCES

Bradshaw J., *Healing the Shame that Binds You*. Health Communications, Inc., Deerfield, FL, 1988.

de Saint Exupery A. *Wind, sand and stars*. Reynolds & Hetchcock, New York, 1939.

Ford D, Gibson P, Dreifuss F. Psychosocial considerations in childhood epilepsy. In *Pediatric Neurology: Classification and Management of Seizures in the Child*, ed. F Dreifuss. John Wright, PSG Inc., Boston, 1983, pp. 277–95.

Goldin G, Margolin R. The psychosocial aspects of epilepsy. In *Epilepsy Rehabilitation*, ed. GN Wright. Little, Brown, Boston, 1975, pp. 66–79.

Hemingway Ernest. *A Farewell to Arms*. Scribner, New York, 1929.

Lechtenberg R. *Epilepsy and the Family*. Harvard Press, Cambridge, MA, 1984.

Lechtenberg R, Akner L. Psychologic adaptation of children to epilepsy in a parent. *Epilepsia* 1984; 25(1):40–5.

Meyer DJ, Vadasy P, Fewell RR. *Living with a Brother or Sister with Special Needs: a Book for Sibs*. University of Washington Press, Seattle, 1985.

Shain M. *When Lovers are Friends*. J.B. Lippincott, New York, 1978.

Trimble M. *Women and Epilepsy*. Wiley, New York, 1991.

Usisken S, Goldin G, Perry S.L. *The Rehabilitation of the Young Epileptic*. Lexington Books, Lexington, MA, 1971.

24

Parenting the daughter with epilepsy

Joan Kessner Austin and Janet Austin Tooze

Epilepsy affects every member of a family. A parent raising a young child with epilepsy has understandable concerns about the child's safety, but also understands that children need to run and climb, to ride a bike, and to swim. As the child grows, the parent decides about play dates, sleepovers, and summer camp. The adolescent wants to drive a car. Protecting and enhancing the child's emotional health are even more of a challenge. Ensuring healthy self-esteem is never easy, but when a child is dealing with a chronic illness, the difficulty is amplified.

Therefore, I felt it was important to include the perspective of a mother and daughter who had successfully dealt with epilepsy. I asked Janet Austin Tooze and her mother Joan Kessner Austin to share their personal experience – particularly how they had placed epilepsy in the proper perspective. I think you will find their story sincere, truthful, and moving. Although epilepsy is no longer part of their day-to-day life, it remains part of their family experience.

Dr Joan Kessner Austin has a PhD in nursing and her research has concerned the impact of chronic illness on the development of children with epilepsy and other chronic medical conditions. Her work has earned her a Javits Award from the National Institutes of Health as well as election to the Institute of Medicine. Janet Austin Tooze is now completing graduate work in statistics and is entering a health research career. Here is a story of how epilepsy affected, but did not define, one mother and daughter.

MJM

I have just hung up the telephone after talking with my daughter, Janet, about her course options in relation to a minor for her PhD program in biostatistics. She has narrowed her choices to courses in either pharmacology or pharmacy. Janet is 28 years old, married, a full-time doctoral student, and working 20 hours a week as a data analyst. She is attractive, competent, and well adjusted. Upon hanging up the telephone I am struck again with just how proud I am of her and all that she has accomplished. As I

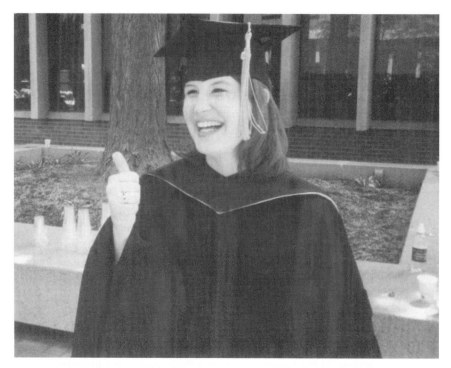

Figure 24.1 Janet Austin Tooze.

look back 22 years to the time when she was diagnosed with epilepsy, I realize how very differently things have turned out from what I had originally feared.

In the preparation of this chapter, I have reflected back on my own experience and asked Janet to reflect on what she remembers and what advice she might have for parents. Over these past two decades, I also have become a nurse researcher who focuses on children with epilepsy and their families. I have learned a great deal about coping with epilepsy from parents who have participated in my research and I incorporate that information into my comments here. Even though this chapter refers to girls, almost all of it should apply to boys. Janet's reminiscences and advice are interspersed throughout the chapter.

As parents, we want our children to grow up to be independent, kind, loving, well educated, and competent. Parenting a healthy daughter can be a challenge under ideal circumstances. When a child develops epilepsy, however, it adds a whole new layer of difficulty to parenting. Seizures are disruptive, especially at the beginning. Janet's seizures were unexpected, unwelcome, and a threat to our hopes and dreams for her.

I still remember being in the doctor's office as I heard the words 'abnormal EEG . . . anticonvulsant . . . epilepsy.' I had to sit down. Somehow, my past nursing education and experience did not help me cope with this new situation. My knees shook uncontrollably. I could hear the doctor talking, but the words he said did not make sense to me. In a way, he was giving me hope, but in another way he was scaring me to death. My worst fear was that my daughter had a brain tumor. The doctor's words slowly registered. Janet did not have a brain tumor. I was afraid to accept it, but, little by little, I nudged this fear aside. However, I still worried about how her life would be affected by the epilepsy.

It took a few days for the full effect of the diagnosis to sink in. I worried about how the seizures would affect her. Would she be able to live a normal life? What would the seizures and the medication do to her brain? Would the medication affect her learning? Then the overriding concern: would Janet be able to live up to her potential? We had known since the first few months of her life how very bright she was. She figured out the children's toy puzzles in record time, was very creative with a crayon and paper, and spoke clearly in full sentences long before children are expected to. I worried, too, about her social development, especially because she had always been a bit shy. How would seizures affect friendships? Would she date? Would she get married? Would she be able to become a healthy mother of her own children?

I knew I had to get over my fears if I was going to be the parent she needed to help her deal with this experience. When I interacted with Janet, I tried to keep my fears from affecting her, but my husband and I could tell that Janet was worried, too. She was only 6 at the time of her first seizures, but she told us later just how frightened she really was.

Janet Reminisces

I was scared during my seizures. I worried that I might die. They happened at night when I was alone in my room. I think the worst part of having seizures was the lack of control I experienced. I would be awakened from sleep by my seizures, and then just have to 'watch' as my left arm and leg jerked uncontrollably. I would yell for my parents, and they would come into my room, but there was really nothing anyone could do. There were times when I felt like I couldn't breathe during my seizures, which just emphasized how out of control I felt.

I remember trying to regain control of my life. I tried to figure out what had caused the seizures. One day, when I was watching TV, it was interrupted by a special announcement about people who had unknowingly been poisoned. I don't remember the details, but the announcement ended with the consequences of poisoning, one of which was having seizures. I hadn't quite grasped the concept of 'cause-and-effect' yet, and I came to the conclusion that all seizures were caused by poisoning and that I must have been poisoned. Because I had my seizures in bed I looked for poison on my pillow. Also, because my seizures started in my left hand, I thought there was poison on my hand. So I began to wash my hands obsessively, trying to get rid of the poison. Of course, what I didn't know was that my seizures were not caused by poisoning. In my 6-year-old mind, I was trying to gain control by getting rid of the seizures.

My seizures were treated with phenobarbital, which has a lot of side effects. As a child, I really didn't understand what having side effects meant. The phenobarbital made me feel as if I were living in a fog, but I didn't realize that I felt that way because of the medicine. I just thought it was me. I'd always be the last one to finish an exam in school, until I went off my medication. I remember the first time I took a test after I quit taking my medication. I was the first one to finish the test, and I was convinced I must have skipped a page or something. Because I had seizures when I started school, I'd always assumed I was just slow. My mother tells me that the new anticonvulsant medications have fewer side effects, so hopefully this is not such a big problem for kids today.

I remember being confused about going to the neurologist. Even when I was 16, and had been seeing one for years, he still didn't seem like a real doctor to me. We would go into his office, and my mom and I would sit in chairs in front of his desk and discuss my treatment. I had always thought of a doctor as someone in a white coat who took your temperature and listened to your chest, not as some guy who wore a sport coat and sat behind a desk and asked you questions.

Things were most difficult for my daughter, my husband, and me at the beginning as we tried to understand and deal with epilepsy. As I look back on it, I was simultaneously trying to juggle three major parenting tasks. First, I was trying to learn as much as I needed to know about epilepsy and handling future seizures so I could take good care of Janet. Second, I was trying to help her deal with having seizures and the side effects of the medication. Third, I was trying to come to terms with what epilepsy was doing to me; I was sad and afraid. I knew I had to handle my own emotions if I were to be able to be effective in helping Janet. The rest of the chapter focuses on these three parenting tasks: learning about epilepsy, helping your daughter, and coming to terms with having a daughter with epilepsy.

Learning about epilepsy

Epilepsy is a chronic condition that will probably be in your life many years and, therefore, it is necessary for you to learn all you can about your child's seizures and treatment. Parents have a lot of responsibility in managing the epilepsy because they are ultimately responsible for their child's health care. They are responsible for buying medication, making sure the medication is taken in the proper manner, and watching for side effects. Parents must decide when to take their child to the doctor for care and when to ask for a second opinion about that care. The only way to do this job properly is to be knowledgeable about your child's seizure condition.

Box 24.1

My advice is to prepare yourself for visits with the doctor and make sure that you leave with the information you need. The best way I know to do that is to go to the visit with questions written down and take the time you need to get your questions answered. Your child should also have an opportunity to ask questions and get them answered at the visits.

Initially, it is essential that you learn how to care for your child's immediate health. Minimally, you need to know what to do when your child has another seizure, how to give the medication, which medication side effects should be reported, and when things are serious enough to call the doctor or take her to the hospital. The physician or nurse in the office should provide you with basic information and direct you to other sources. (If they have not told you, let me be the first to recommend the Epilepsy Foundation of America as a source of accurate information.) You need to go to office visits prepared to obtain the information you need. Ask your doctor specific questions so you will be very clear about what you need to do. For example, questions you might want to ask are:

- 'What should I do when my daughter has another seizure?'
- 'At what point would I need to take her to the hospital?'
- 'How long does it take for the medication to work?'
- 'What should I do if she misses a dose or is sick with the flu and can't keep anything in her stomach?'
- 'What medication side effects are serious and mean that my daughter should be taken off the medication?'
- 'Which side effects do I not need to worry about?'

Getting what you need from an office visit is a task that neither I nor parents in my research studies handled easily. One problem for me was that I was afraid to show my ignorance, particularly because I was a nurse and should know better. Another problem was that I was overly concerned about taking up too much of the doctor's time. For example, if the doctor was late, I would try to be quicker. I am not sure why the doctor's time was such a worry to me, but I have had many parents tell me they do the same thing. My advice is to prepare yourself for visits with the doctor and make sure that you leave with the information you need. The best way I know to do that is to go to the visit with questions written down and take the time you need to get your questions answered. Your child should also have an opportunity to ask questions and get them answered at the visits.

Another way to learn about epilepsy is to read books written specifically for parents, although parents find it difficult to learn about their own child's epilepsy from books because most books cover the entire field of epilepsy. Because epilepsy refers to recurrent seizures, it covers a whole host of diverse conditions that cause seizures. Sometimes, epilepsy is very mild, with seizures that are easily controlled. At other times, epilepsy is very serious and has associated learning and behavior problems. Reading a book that covers everything can be confusing because you may not be sure exactly which parts apply to your child's condition. Learning about complicated cases can also be frightening because it brings up problems you did not even know existed. At the beginning, when I was so frightened, I avoided reading general materials on epilepsy for fear that I might read about something that would make me even more worried. Later, when I was more comfortable with the nature of Janet's seizures, I found reading these books to be helpful. My advice is to read the books but keep in mind that they cover a great deal of information that may or may not apply to your child's condition.

Box 24.2

It is probably a good idea to keep a seizure diary, including missed doses and other illnesses, where you can write all of this information down and take it with you to the doctor's visit. Keeping this information may also help you notice seizure patterns and perhaps provide clues as to measures that may decrease the frequency of seizures or make them less severe.

Another thing that may make it difficult to learn about your child's seizures is that some questions cannot be definitively answered by anyone. For example, in about two-thirds of cases there is no certain answer as to why a child developed seizures. I worried that perhaps I was at fault. When there is no known cause for the seizures, it is easy to imagine the worst and believe you might have done something to cause them. One way to handle this guilt is to write down what you are worried about and ask the doctor whether your actions could have caused the seizures. Even though there might not be definite answers in all cases, at least obtaining the information that some events probably did not cause the seizures should reduce the number of things about which you are worrying or feeling guilty.

Another important source of learning comes from your own observations of your child's seizures. As a parent, you play an important role in describing your child's seizures to the doctor, because you are the one most likely to see the seizures. It is important that you report relevant information back to the doctor because descriptions of seizures can help with the diagnosis and treatment of the epilepsy. Doctors are interested in knowing what the seizure looked like, what your child was doing immediately before it began, what you noticed first, what happened second, what happened third, how long the seizure lasted, and how long it took for your child to return to normal. It is probably a good idea to keep a seizure diary, including missed doses and other illnesses, where you can write all of this information down and take it with you to the doctor's visit. Keeping this information may also help you notice seizure patterns and perhaps provide clues as to measures that may decrease the frequency of seizures or make them less severe.

Helping your daughter

The onset of Janet's seizures was quite stressful. Her first seizure was followed within minutes by two more. After the second seizure, we made a hurried trip to the hospital emergency room. Adding to the stress was the fact that she did not lose consciousness during the seizures and, because of this, she was worried that she would suffocate. The seizures affected the whole left side of her body and greatly restricted her breathing. Understandably, she was worried about suffocating.

Despite this stressful beginning, seizures did not turn out to be a major problem for Janet. Over the course of about 3 years, she had about 30 more seizures and then became seizure free. She stopped taking medication in early adolescence and has been seizure free ever since. Our experience is similar to that of many other families. In our research studies, about half of the children become seizure free and are able to stop taking their medication. My research also shows that, even when children do not outgrow epilepsy, most of them and their families adapt well. Nevertheless, even though it might be reassuring to know that most children do well in time, that does not mean that children do not need help in dealing with the epilepsy in the meantime.

One of the first tasks in helping your daughter is to explore her feelings about having seizures. In our studies we find children to have many fears and concerns, though very often these worries are unfounded. For example, many children worry about dying when the chance of that is extremely low. Therefore, it is important to talk with your daughter and find out what she is worrying about so that you can help her cope realistically with these worries. Sometimes it is difficult to talk about things that are uncomfortable. There might be a tendency not to bring up the topic at all because it is stressful. However, in the long term it will be much less stressful for you and your daughter if she can tell you what she is feeling. Once concerns are out in the open, you can help her develop strategies for dealing with them. Sometimes, just knowing the facts about epilepsy can be very reassuring. Involve your child as much as possible with doctors' visits and bring questions to be answered. Worries need to be addressed and they should not be swept under the rug.

In our studies many children have also told us that they are afraid they might be injured during a seizure. Some seizures are so fleeting that the chances of getting hurt are almost nonexistent. With most other seizure types, the chances are still rare. If your child has a seizure type that could result in injury, it is important to teach the people she is in contact with how to administer first aid.

Many children with epilepsy have social concerns. In our research we find adolescent girls to be especially concerned with their appearance and social acceptance. The teenagers in our studies also report that they worry about telling others about their seizures and need help in deciding how to do it. Other children have told us they worry about having a seizure in front of their peers and being teased. That is a very real concern. Children can be very cruel to children who are different. Dealing with teasing is not easy for children or for parents. When Janet was teased about having seizures, it was difficult for me not to call the parents of the child who teased her and tell them off. I wanted to, but I decided it would not really be helpful. It is important for children to fit in and be accepted by their peers. The last thing they want is to be different, and having seizures can make some children feel different. If your child is having problems with friends, it might be helpful to do whatever you can to support their friendships with other children. Be the agreeable parent. Make your home inviting for other children. If parents are open to other children, their children will have more friends. Encourage group activities, such as Girl Scouts, 4-H, church and school activities, sport teams, dancing lessons, piano lessons, karate, swimming, and pet sitting.

Do not treat your child as if she is different. That can send the message that she is damaged goods or a fragile flower. Being overprotective or over-restricting can also relay the message of fragility. If you feel uncomfortable with your child participating in some activities, it might be helpful to limit the duration of any restriction. For example, you might limit overnights away from home within the first weeks after seizure onset and the initiation of medication. By limiting the restriction to 2 weeks, it sets up a time when things can be re-evaluated. Two weeks later, when you have more information about your child's seizure pattern and response to medication, the restrictions can be reconsidered. Time-limited restrictions should help prevent negative patterns of overprotection and over-restrictions. Another way to prevent your child from feeling different is to avoid overemphasizing the possible effects of the epilepsy. Be straightforward about epilepsy, the same way you are about other health issues, and try not to imagine the worst.

Knowing who and when to tell about the condition is an individual decision for each family. Many things need to be taken into consideration, such as the seizure type, frequency, and severity. Inform people on a need-to-know basis. In my daughter's case, we told selected people when she first experienced seizures and most people handled the information appropriately. We only had problems with a few people. For example, one teacher became very worried and wanted to have a padded tongue blade in the classroom. We finally convinced her that this was not necessary.

As Janet went into middle school and her seizures were under control, she no longer wanted us to tell people. I thought we were doing the right thing at the time because that was what she wanted. A few years ago, however, she told me that she wished she could have been more open about the fact that she had seizures. She said hiding it was probably not a good thing in the long term because it was stressful hiding something about herself. She felt that hiding her seizures made her feel bad about herself. There are no easy answers about dealing with the stigma of epilepsy. All you can do is try to make the best decision at the time and be flexible enough to change strategies as things change. Every child's experience is different. Sometimes it helps to talk to other families to see how they have handled problems.

Overall, I think it is important to talk about epilepsy, but at the same time not to let epilepsy be the main focus of interactions between you and your child. Many parents tell us that one of the most helpful things was to focus on what was normal in their child. I also found that de-emphasizing the seizures and emphasizing the normal was helpful in dealing with Janet's seizures. Keep in mind that most children and their families cope well with seizures and do not have major problems. It also should be encouraging to know that most children's seizures are well controlled and the majority of children enter adulthood with their seizures long behind them.

Janet Reminisces

I don't know many people who would say that they had a 'normal' childhood. Although we tend to think of childhood as a carefree time, many children have to cope with chronic illnesses such as epilepsy, asthma, and allergies. Others must cope with cancer and other serious illnesses and others have to deal with the psychological stress associated with divorce or even child abuse. Even children who manage to escape illnesses or other stresses are teased by other children for one reason or another. Fortunately, children can be extremely brave and resilient when dealing with these problems. And they do grow up to be 'normal' adults.

Most of my classmates did not know that I had epilepsy. When I was in the fifth grade one boy, who was at the orthodontist the same time I was, overheard the dentist talking to me about my seizures and later, at school, teased me about having epilepsy. He stumbled over the word, putting too many 's's in it. I laughed and said, 'You can't even pronounce it.' I sounded cool, but I felt ashamed. After that experience, I definitely didn't want anyone else at school to find out.

When I was living in a dorm my freshman year of college, a girl slipped coming out of the shower, hit her head, and had a seizure. I realized there was nothing that I could do while it was happening, except wait. Afterwards, I told her that I had had seizures as a child. That experience influenced me to tell another friend my most secret of secrets. I worked slowly up to the point, but when I had finished she said, 'That's it?' She'd been expecting something important. Now I'm comfortable sharing with people if the subject comes up. Surprisingly, they don't see it as a big deal. To them, I am the same person I always have been. It was a good feeling to realize that I was accepted by people for who I was, and no longer had to be scared to share with others that I once had epilepsy. This made me think that perhaps I should have told people sooner, but perhaps as a child I would have been teased had my classmates known about my epilepsy. Dealing with taking my medicine and being worried about seizures along with the everyday pressures of childhood was enough for me at that time. I really did not want to have to deal with the extra teasing that probably would have gone along with the other kids knowing I was 'different.'

Coming to terms with having a daughter with epilepsy

Although it might be reassuring to know that most families do well, it does not take away from the fact that you need to adjust to having a child with a chronic health condition. Finding yourself in the situation of raising a daughter with epilepsy is stressful, especially at the beginning. Part of the reason is that parents put their own worries, fears, and feelings on the back burner so they can concentrate on getting their child the care and support she needs. Coming to terms with epilepsy takes time. Good health is at the top of the list of all the things we want for our children, and epilepsy is a threat to this strong desire. The course of epilepsy is often unpredictable; parents have no way to predict how long or severely epilepsy will affect their child. Furthermore, there is still a stigma associated with epilepsy that makes it more difficult to talk to others about it. Parents often feel disappointment, anger, and sadness, especially at the beginning when they are just realizing the effects that epilepsy might have on their child's life.

It is hard to accept the fact that your child has epilepsy, but that is what you must learn to do. Most of the coping involves coming to terms with epilepsy on an emotional level. You cannot stop the seizures. All you can do is to get your child the best treatment possible and make sure that you are giving the medication as ordered. After that, you just have to deal with your feelings. As adults, we have experience coping with things we do not like and cannot change. I tried to apply those same coping strategies to dealing with Janet's epilepsy. All of us use different methods for dealing with strong negative feelings. In our case, my husband and I used different, and at times conflicting, strategies. I found it helpful to talk about my concerns and my husband appeared to be avoiding the subject. At first, I was angry with him, not only because I thought he was not dealing with it, but because he was thwarting my coping efforts. What I did not know at the time was that he was dealing with it internally and my talking about my concerns and fears made him more anxious. At the beginning, I found support from friends and family. Over time, my husband and I were better able to support each other.

My research has convinced me that one of the most important things parents can do is to develop an optimistic attitude. Personally, it was helpful for me to focus on the positive things about the situation and not on the fact that I did not want my daughter to have seizures. For example, I would tell myself that we were getting the best care possible, that most children did well, and that she did not have a brain tumor. I also actively stopped myself from dwelling on all of the possible problems that could arise from the seizures.

In our research studies we have found that parents as well as children have concerns that are based on incomplete or inaccurate information. Sometimes, simply obtaining more specific information about your child's seizure condition can help reduce worry. For example, I really did not need to worry about a brain tumor being missed because the clinical examination and tests would have given clues to that effect. Today, there are newer and even better techniques to uncover brain tumors. To reduce stress, write down your fears and concerns and go over them with the doctor or nurse. Many of them probably will be unfounded. If they are possible problems, find out what you should do to prevent them. For example, some children with seizure conditions do have problems with school work. In this case, get psychological and achievement testing and plan to have additional help for your daughter at the first sign of problems. Starting tutoring before problems escalate is a good strategy, no matter what the source of the problem.

Some parents say that talking to other parents whose children also have epilepsy has been helpful to them. They learned they were not alone and they learned how other families handled similar problems. Because epilepsy is so diverse, it is especially helpful to talk to parents whose children are similar in age and who have similar types of seizures. Otherwise, their experience may be very different from yours and their solutions not applicable to your problems.

Sometimes, especially at the beginning, parents change the way they discipline or react to their child with epilepsy. Our studies indicate that children watch how their parents are behaving to try to work out what is going on. Therefore, it is important that you keep parenting rules such as discipline as normal as possible. That does not mean that you might not watch your child more closely for a while, but keep things in perspective. It is important that children are not over-restricted and it is important to learn just what restrictions, if any, are necessary. Instituting appropriate safety precautions can minimize the need for restrictions. Whenever possible, it is important that children do the same things they were doing before the seizures. Sometimes, we are tempted to indulge our daughters a bit to try to make up for the fact that they are having to deal with this difficult condition. I know that I did this for a while with Janet. However, being overprotective and overindulgent in the long term gives them the message that they are different. When a child is treated like a fragile flower, she can get the message that she is weak.

Janet's Advice

Having epilepsy did affect who I am today. I'm sure of that. But so did being in Girl Scouts and 4-H, and moving from Texas to Indiana between the second and third grades. One of the biggest influences on my life was having a mother who believed that girls could excel in math and science, and encouraged me in those areas as well as being a role model for me. I guess what I'm trying to say is that having epilepsy influenced who I am today, but it did not define me. I used to think epilepsy was vastly important. For a while it was. But now it is just something that I went through a long time ago – like wearing braces. It's part of who I am, but only a small part. There are many people who did not outgrow epilepsy and who didn't allow it to keep them from pursuing their goals and dreams; I don't think anyone should. A poster that hangs in my mother's office sums it up best: 'A person with epilepsy is a *person* who just happens to have epilepsy.' It's important to focus on your daughter's spiritual, physical, and emotional well-being, not just the part of her brain that's causing her seizures.

I know that my parents talked to me about having epilepsy, but I'm not sure if they realized how little I really understood. I would advise parents to really talk to their kids about their epilepsy and make sure they really understand how naive children can be about things. Continue these conversations over the years, because children are able to understand things more deeply as they mature. Talk to them about epilepsy and what it is. Let them know that there's nothing they can do to stop it, but they can help keep it under control if they take their medication. Let them know that you're always there for them if they have any questions about their epilepsy and that, even though you may not know the answers, you can find them out together. Explain to them how a neurologist is different from their pediatrician, and that everyone who goes to a neurologist doesn't have epilepsy. And after you go to the doctor, discuss what he or she said and what it means.

I think it is also important for parents to remember that children face new challenges every day. I think that dealing with epilepsy, for a child, is just one of those challenges. No one would choose to have epilepsy, but everyone can choose how to respond to it. My advice to a parent would be to view your child as you would if she didn't have epilepsy – as a young person who is discovering life, planning her future, and realizing her full potential.

Postscript

By the way, Janet decided to minor in pharmacology.

25

Safety issues for women with epilepsy

Patricia Dean

Health-care providers caring for people with epilepsy generally have the same goals. Those goals are to stop seizures, avoid treatment-related side effects, and ensure a good quality of life. Ideally, no one's life would be significantly changed because of epilepsy. People with epilepsy are usually counseled to take advantage of usual life experiences. On the other hand, some precautions may be necessary, depending on the type of seizures and seizure frequency.

In this chapter, Patricia Dean discusses reasonable safety measures for people with epilepsy to consider. Pat is an Epilepsy Nurse Specialist. Her professional life has focused on the care of people with epilepsy and she is currently at the University of Miami. Pat is also on the Board of Directors of the National Epilepsy Foundation and is President of her local Epilepsy Foundation affiliate, Epilepsy Foundation of South Florida. She provides a reasonable and complete discussion of the risks related to seizures and offers suggestions to ensure seizure safety while leading a full and active life.

MJM

A number of published medical studies have examined whether people with epilepsy are at risk for injuries as a result of seizures. Although some studies conclude that there is no higher risk of injury for people with epilepsy than for the general population, other studies suggest that people with seizures are at greater risk (Hauser et al., 1984). For example, injuries are most likely to occur in people with frequent seizures and in those whose seizures are associated with loss of consciousness or loss of motor control, particularly tonic–clonic or atonic seizures.

In general, women and men are at equal risk for injury during a seizure. However, women are twice as likely as men to be burned or scalded during a seizure. This is probably because women are more likely to be cooking, ironing, and handling hot objects such as hair dryers and curling irons.

Childbearing and, for the most part, child rearing are the province of women. Although pregnant women with epilepsy are often concerned that a seizure may cause injury to themselves and their unborn baby, there are no studies that specifically evaluate seizure-related injuries during pregnancy. Until recently, women with epilepsy have received little or no education on safely caring for a child. Women with epilepsy were told for many years (and some are still being told) not to have children because they would not be able to care for them safely. Although there is no information indicating that the children of women with epilepsy are more likely to be injured, each woman's situation must be individually examined to determine whether a child would be unsafe during a seizure. It was reported that two infants had head trauma when their mothers had myoclonic seizures (brief, lightning-like jerks) during nighttime feedings. In both cases, education about the possible risks to the babies and simple preventative steps (such as feeding while sitting on the floor) could probably have prevented these injuries.

Many seizure-related injuries are preventable. It is important that women are aware of the steps they can take to reduce the risk of injury and how they can live safely with seizures.

Assessing risks

There are many different types of epilepsy. Some people need to make minor adjustments to their lives because of epilepsy, whereas others must make significant life changes. The first step is to decide what risks are posed by seizures in that individual, which can be assessed by asking the following questions.

- *What is the seizure type and how often do seizures occur?* If seizures are frequent, impair consciousness, and affect control of movement, there is a risk that injury will occur.
- *Has a seizure caused injury before?* For example, if a woman has had seizures at work and has injured herself by hitting her head on the corner of her desk, she can have the sharp edges padded to prevent seizure injuries. Evaluating the kind of injury and the situation in which it occurred can reduce or prevent injury next time.

- *Are there seizure patterns or seizure-provoking factors?* Some women have more frequent seizures at certain times of the menstrual cycle. Others have seizures when sleep deprived, when exercising strenuously, or when ill with a cold or flu. If this is the case, 'high-risk' activities, such as a ski trip, can be planned at a time when seizures are less likely to occur. One way to keep track of seizures is to maintain a seizure diary. This is a great tool for helping people to plan their activities as it enables them to know those times when they are more likely to have a seizure. Other ways to help prevent injury are to be aware of whether there is a warning before the seizure. When seizures begin with an aura (simple partial seizure), this may give a person time to get to a safe place or position.
- *Am I safe if I had a seizure while doing this?* Can this activity be made safer for someone with seizures? Asking herself these questions is another possible way for a woman to prevent injury. For example, turning the temperature down on the hot water heater may prevent scalding during bathing or a shower. Cooking on a microwave may be preferred over cooking on a stove (see Table 25.1 for additional home safety tips).

Workplace issues and epilepsy

In the past, it has not always been easy for women to advance in the workplace and many women with epilepsy fear that their condition may prevent them from getting jobs for which they are well qualified or that they may be unable to obtain promotions. Because of the stigma associated with epilepsy, many people struggle with the issue of whether or not to disclose their condition. It is important to note that a person with epilepsy, according to the Americans with Disabilities Act, is not required by law to disclose his or her epilepsy prior to a job offer or to disclose it at all unless it is relevant to the job.

Regardless of whether or not a woman chooses to disclose that she has epilepsy, there are a few things she should keep in mind while at work. It is important to review any job-related risks and assess whether something can be changed to improve safety. If a woman feels comfortable, she might consider telling her coworkers that she has epilepsy and educating them on the correct first aid for seizures. If a woman is working in what is considered a nontraditional job, she should climb only as high as she can safely fall,

Table 25.1. Safety tips at homes

To prevent burn injuries when using running water, set the temperature low so that you will not
be scalded if you lose consciousness. Always turn the cold water on first. If sensation is a problem,
ask someone to check the water temperature for you.

Use a microwave oven for cooking or remove burner controls from gas or electric stoves when
not in use. When cooking on a stove, try to use the back burners as much as possible.

Serve hot foods or liquids directly from stoves or countertops onto plates.

Slide containers of hot food along the counter instead of picking them up, or use a cart when
taking hot foods or liquids from one spot to another. Even better, let someone else carry
them. Cook when someone else is in the house when possible. If you are alone, consider eating
cold foods, order a food delivery, or eat out.

When drinking hot liquids such as coffee or tea, use a cup with a lid to prevent burns from spills.

Cover heating units and put guards around fireplaces.

Avoid cigarette smoking.

Avoid ironing when alone and use irons with automatic shut-off. Buy clothes that do not need
ironing whenever possible.

Curling irons and hair dryers can cause burns during a seizure. If used, make sure the curling iron
has an automatic shut-off switch. Use the hair dryer on a cool setting rather than a hot one.

Avoid space heaters, particularly in small spaces such as bathrooms. If a heater is used, place it at
a good distance from where you stand or sit.

Other kitchen tips

Use pre-cut or already prepared foods as much as possible. Use a blender or food processor rather
than a sharp knife.

Wear rubber gloves when handling knives or washing dishes and glassware in the sink.

Use plastic rather than glass containers as much as possible.

Store all frequently used items at accessible heights.

---

especially on a concrete floor, unless she is protected by a reliable safety
harness and wearing a secure hard hat or helmet. When a woman with
epilepsy is working with machinery, safety features should be checked, such
as automatic shut-offs or safety guards. If she is sensitive to flashing lights,
she can try to limit her exposure, look away if possible, or wear dark glasses.

Although it can be difficult, a woman with epilepsy should try to keep
consistent work hours so she does not have to go a long time without sleep
(see Chapter 2). It is important to evaluate whether or not stress makes her

seizures worse. If a woman has a high-stress job that demands long working hours, she should find ways to reduce stress on the job (Epilepsy Foundation, 2000).

Personal safety, women, and violence

We live in a world in which acts of violence against women are almost commonplace. According to the United States Justice Department, women are the victims of more than 4.5 million violent crimes each year, including approximately 500 000 rapes or sexual assaults.

All women have to worry about personal safety to some degree. Although there is no real evidence that women with epilepsy are at a higher risk of becoming victims of crime, a recent informal survey conducted by the Epilepsy Foundation raises concern. In this survey of 245 women with epilepsy between the ages of 16 and 82, 20% stated that being assaulted in any way during a seizure was at least sometimes a problem for them. It is difficult to know from this survey whether these women were concerned about violence or had actually been victims of violence. Whether or not the respondents to the survey were victims of violence, this is an important issue for many women with epilepsy.

Law enforcement personnel often speak to women about ways to avoid becoming a victim of crime. Women are often counseled not to walk alone at night in certain areas, and are encouraged to stay alert, to be wary of strangers, and to have car keys in their hand when going into an empty parking garage alone.

Maintaining personal safety is crucial for all women with epilepsy. For many, parenting and maintaining a household raise additional safety concerns. Certain adjustments in the environment and in daily routines can minimize the risk of injury from seizures. By working together with health-care professionals, women with epilepsy and their families can better understand their seizures, assess work and home situations, and make the adjustments necessary to manage epilepsy and lead an interesting and productive life. Health-care providers must be supportive and help women find an appropriate balance between safe, healthy behaviors and personal goals and desired quality of life.

SELECTED REFERENCES

Annegers J, Grabow J, Groover R, Laws E, Elveback L, Kurland L. Seizures after head trauma: a population study. *Neurology* 1980; 30:683–9.

Bachman R, Saltzman L. Violence against women: estimates from the redesigned survey. Department of Justice Estimates, Annapolis Junction, MD, 1995.

Buck D, Baker G, Jacoby A, Smith D, Chadwick D. Patients' experiences of injury as a result of epilepsy. *Epilepsia* 1997; 38(4):439–44.

Dean P, Duchowny M, Harvey AS. Epileptic head injury by-proxy in maternal juvenile myoclonic epilepsy masquerading as child abuse. *Epilepsia* 1995; 36(Suppl. 4):100.

Hauser W, Tabaddor K, Factor P, Finer C. Seizures and head injury in an urban community. *Neurology* 1984; 34:746–51.

Osborne Shafer P, Austin D, Callanan M, Clerico C. Safety and activities of daily living for people with epilepsy. In *Managing Seizure Disorders*, ed. N Santilli. Lippincott-Raven, Philadelphia, 1996, pp. 1151–9.

Pennell, P. *Epilepsy and Pregnancy*. Epilepsy Foundation of America Annual Meeting, 1997.

Safety and Seizures. Epilepsy Foundation of America, Landover, MD, 1996.

Safety Tips – Daily Living and Workplace Safety; Safety and Seizures: Tips for Living with Seizure Disorders. Epilepsy Foundation, Landover, MD, 1996.

Spitz M, Towbin J, Shantz D, Adler L. Risk factors for burns as a consequence of seizures in persons with epilepsy. *Epilepsia* 1994; 35(4):764–7.

26

Legal issues facing women with epilepsy

Jeanne Carpenter

Jeanne Carpenter is a partner in a Washington-based law firm. She is past President and Chair of the Epilepsy Foundation and is currently on the National Board of Directors. She is an eloquent spokesperson on behalf of people with epilepsy and has been a strong supporter of the Epilepsy Foundation's Women with Epilepsy Initiative. As a woman with epilepsy, Ms Carpenter has experienced many of the challenges discussed in this book. In this chapter she addresses the legal issues of importance to women with epilepsy. These include employment, motor vehicle licensing, family law, and insurance.

MJM

Introduction

I was diagnosed with epilepsy when I was in my mid-twenties. After I heard my physician's view about the possible physical restrictions I would confront because of my seizures and the possible side effects of the medications, my immediate questions turned to how others might limit me and my daily activities. Could I still drive? Would my epilepsy impact my new job as an attorney? Did I have to disclose my epilepsy when making various types of applications? Would my medical insurance cover my doctor and hospital bills? These are common questions among women diagnosed with epilepsy and many raise possible legal issues that are not unique to women.

This chapter summarizes many of the areas in which legal issues arise; it is not intended to provide legal advice, nor can all legal issues that may result from epilepsy be answered, but it attempts to outline major issues for the most common concerns among those of us with epilepsy. If, after reading this chapter or any of the references listed at the end of it, you have a legal question or believe you have some type of claim, the best course of action is to contact an attorney who specializes in employment discrimination or

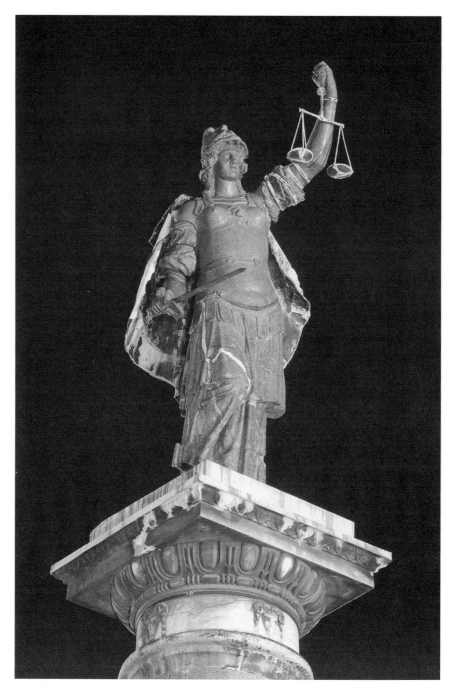

Figure 26.1 Themis, the Goddess of Justice.

other representation of the disabled. Attorney references can be obtained from your local Epilepsy Foundation affiliate, the national Foundation office, or your local bar association. The Epilepsy Foundation also has excellent summaries of various legal issues, including a handbook on the Americans With Disabilities Act.

Employment

Usually, when a women is diagnosed with epilepsy or reaches the age of permanent employment, her first questions will focus on whether her epilepsy will affect how she is employed and promoted, the type of job she can obtain, or the likelihood that she will successfully apply for the type of position she seeks. In the last few years, a potent tool has been in place with Congress' passage in 1990 of the Americans With Disabilities Act (ADA). In short, the ADA prohibits most employers from discriminating on the basis of disability if the applicant or the employee is able to perform the job's essential functions. The ADA also prohibits discrimination in the activities of state and local governments, public and private transportation, public accommodations, and telecommunications.

The purpose and intent of the statute were to ensure that those with a disability enjoyed protection against discrimination. As with any new statute, many of the cases that have been brought under the ADA, including those filed by individuals with epilepsy, have not resulted in relief for the plaintiff because the facts of the case have not been developed and alleged in a manner that the court has found would sustain a cause of action. However, with more lawyers understanding the important elements of the statute and what one most show in order successfully to claim discrimination due to one's disability, the use of the statute will only increase. To the extent that those who must comply with the statute also understand its requirements and the threat of successful litigation against them, the extent of voluntary compliance with the law will increase.

Overview of the ADA as it relates to employment

The employment provisions of the ADA provide that 'no covered entity shall discriminate against a qualified individual with a disability because of the disability in regard to discharge of employees and other terms, conditions and privileges of employment.' In order to establish a claim, an individual must prove that he or she: (1) has a disability; (2) is a 'qualified' individual; and (3) was discriminated against because of the disability by the employer in the firing or other condition of employment. The decisions of many courts have devoted substantial analysis and explanation to the nature and scope of these requirements, each of which is briefly summarized here.

Disability

In order to claim a 'disability' under the ADA, an individual must have either a physical or mental impairment that substantially limits one or more of his or her life activities, have a record of this impairment, or be regarded as having such impairment. Many cases have discussed whether epilepsy or seizure disorders qualify as such a disability. Because of the variety of types of seizures and the manner in which they manifest themselves, the definition of epilepsy as a disability for purposes of the ADA has not been clear in all instances. However, many courts have concluded that even partial seizures can properly classify someone as having a disability because, in the absence of medication, an individual would be unable to partake in major life activities such as walking, seeing, hearing, speaking, breathing, learning, or working. Therefore, at least one court has held that the fact that an individual has not actually had a seizure for several months because of the successful control by medication would not preclude claiming a disability under the ADA. Generally, the establishment of epilepsy as a disability is the easiest element of the ADA case to satisfy.

Qualified individual

One of the keystones of the ADA is that the individual with the disability must be qualified in order to maintain a claim. Employers are not required to modify the prerequisites for an individual job in order to customize the position for the individual with the disability, e.g., educational or other types of objective qualifications need not be changed. The individual with a disability must be able to perform the 'essential functions' of the position, an ability that is frequently challenged by employers defending against ADA lawsuits brought by individuals with epilepsy. If the employee cannot perform the job's essential functions, the ADA requires the employer to make 'reasonable accommodation' to permit the disabled employee to complete the job's tasks.

The line between what constitutes an essential function of a job, on one hand, and an unreasonable or overly burdensome required accommodation, on the other, can sometimes be quite difficult to discern. For example, individuals with epilepsy may be denied certain jobs because driving (and, therefore, the possession of a driver's license) was considered an essential function of the position, e.g., a delivery service. In a recent hotly contested case, an individual with epilepsy who was discharged from his position as a shoe store sales clerk was found by a court to be unable to perform the essential function of safeguarding the store and its goods during the time that he suffered from a seizure. Whether a particular aspect of a job position is actually a convenience or truly is an 'essential function' can be a subject of tremendous debate and argument during the course of a claim or case under the ADA.

Similarly, the validity under the ADA of an accommodation that is either proposed as reasonable by an employer or sought as an alternative by an employee creates controversy and disagreement. The employer and court must ask and evaluate whether modification of work facilities, job restructuring, a change in work schedule, or other such accommodation is reasonable or an alteration of the essential functions of the job. The accommodations required by the ADA are not without limitation, but must merely be considered 'reasonable.'

A recent appellate court decision held that the ADA did not require an employer to sacrifice the provisions of a union collective bargaining agreement in order to provide the accommodation requested by a railroad worker with epilepsy who could no longer work alone at heights or operate dangerous machinery. The worker had requested reassignment from the railroad by invoking a provision of the collective bargaining agreement that allowed him, as a disabled employee, to be assigned to a position occupied by a more senior employee if he was capable of performing the job duties. The railway refused, fearing that the union contract would be endangered, and offered an alternative accommodation in the form of an escort on the stairs. The court agreed that this was a reasonable accommodation and that the employer need not be forced to select the best such alternative available, i.e., the assignment to a different position.

Similarly, in another case, a court held that a cleaning crew employee with epilepsy was not discriminated against when his employer refused to provide him with free transportation to a new cleaning site and also refused a change in work schedule because the job had a specific completion time. The court found that the employee had either walked, biked, or taken a bus to earlier jobs that were only half a mile closer to his home and had never adequately explained why he required a more extensive accommodation at this new cleaning site.

As these cases illustrate, the finding as to whether an employer has made a reasonable accommodation frequently turns on the facts of an individual case and on the good faith of the employer in proposing an alternative to the disabled employee.

Discrimination based upon the disability

Finally, the negative or adverse employment action, whether it is demotion or termination, must constitute unlawful discrimination on the basis of the disability. The purpose of this element of the ADA is to forbid discrimination that is based on stereotypical conduct or beliefs, by which individuals with epilepsy are frequently victimized. Instead, the ADA requires that an employee's ability to do his or her job be analyzed on an individualized, demonstrable basis.

Procedures under the ADA

If a woman believes she has been discriminated against because she has epilepsy, she may file a claim with the Equal Employment Opportunity Commission (EEOC) within 180 days of the action of which she complains, e.g., the dismissal or demotion. The EEOC will undertake an investigation of the allegations made in the claim and, if it determines that reasonable grounds exist to believe that discrimination occurred, will undertake resolution through mediation or some other conciliatory process. If such a conciliation is unsuccessful, the EEOC can determine to file a lawsuit in federal court on the woman's behalf or advise her of her right to file suit herself when it issues her a 'right to sue' letter.

Under the ADA, if a claim is successfully pursued either with the EEOC or in federal court, a woman can be awarded equitable relief, such as job reinstatement, back pay and benefits, and a previously denied reasonable accommodation, such as a modification in work schedule. Punitive damages may also be available if the claimant can demonstrate that the discrimination occurred with 'malice or reckless indifference to federally protected rights.' However, certain dollar limitations apply to the award of damages under the ADA.

As with all the legal issues discussed in this chapter, a woman who believes she has been discriminated against should consult a local attorney specializing in discrimination law. In addition, her state may have its own employment discrimination statute that may provide the same or similar types of relief against employment discrimination on behalf of the disabled. Typically, a state's Employment Commission or Department of Labor should be able to provide guidance on the issue.

Other employment issues and statutes

In addition to concerns regarding termination or lack of promotion, a woman with epilepsy may have other concerns about her employment. Although many women with epilepsy do not disclose the fact of their condition while they are applying for jobs because of the fear of rejection, it is unlawful in most instances under the ADA for an employer to ask an applicant whether he or she suffers from epilepsy. Exceptions would include working conditions in which seizures would be a 'direct threat' to the health or safety of the individual or other workers in the vicinity. The ADA requires that these circumstances be evaluated on an individual basis and, except in situations such as transportation positions (e.g., commercial airline pilots), a diagnosis of epilepsy would rarely constitute a direct threat to private or public safety so as to justify any type of job application question or screening.

Unfortunately, the ADA does not cover all employees and employers. Only employers with 15 or more employees are subject to the ADA; however, another federal anti-discrimination statute, the Rehabilitation Act of 1973, or state law may apply. The Rehabilitation Act applies to an employer that is a federal agency, has contracts with the federal government over a certain amount, or receives federal financial assistance.

Driver licensing and reporting

To most women and men in the USA, one of the privileges we take most for granted is our license to drive after we are declared sufficiently capable by the state or other licensing authority. Most states impose a requirement upon those reporting a condition of seizures or epilepsy that we must be seizure free for a designated period, such as 1 year. However, because of the enormous variety in types of seizures, particularly complex partial seizures, many states have re-evaluated the validity of this requirement and instead may look to a variety of other factors in analyzing the capability of a driver with epilepsy. For example, a state may examine whether an individual has a warning or 'aura' prior to the onset of a seizure, whether seizures occur during a customary time of day or month, or whether they tend to have a predictable frequency.

Many states now look to the physician to provide subjective evaluation as to whether an individual should be licensed. Even states with a time-specific period of seizure-free activity may permit an exception if the applicant provides a physician's statement that he or she is appropriately licensed to drive.

When applying for a driver's license, each state asks an applicant whether he or she suffers from a variety of medical conditions, including epilepsy or a seizure disorder. The applicant should answer these questions accurately and truthfully, because the failure to do so could affect his or her liability and insurance coverage in the event of an accident. However, when you apply for a license or a license renewal, it is always wise to take your physician's statement as to your capability to drive, even if you meet your state's seizure-free requirements. In this way, the state is informed as to your neurologist or physician's analysis and will have that letter on file in the event of questions arising in the future.

If have any questions about your particular state's requirements with respect to driver licensing and reporting, the Epilepsy Foundation home page (www.epilepsyfoundation.org) provides a useful, up-to-date summary of information about each state. In addition, you can contact your local Epilepsy Foundation affiliate or the Department of Motor Vehicles in your state to determine the relevant requirements or restrictions applicable to epilepsy prior to applying for or renewing your driver's license.

Child custody and other family issues

For women with epilepsy in particular, the issue of whether they will be able to keep a child in a custody battle, or even adopt a child, is the legal issue that may cause greatest concern. Like the determination to issue a driver's license, states and courts have decided more consistently that it is critical to look behind the type of seizure to evaluate accurately and adequately its impact on the quality of child-rearing. Once again, the statement or testimony of the treating physician or neurologist is critical.

For example, the severity of the seizure disorder, the frequency of occurrence of seizures, their predictability, the length of warning time or 'aura' a woman may experience, and a variety of other factors may contribute to a court's analysis that a woman is capable of maintaining custody of a child notwithstanding a seizure disorder. In fact, several court cases have now established the principle that a seizure disorder or a diagnosis of epilepsy should not be considered the exclusive factor upon which denial of custody can be maintained. In other words, its impact on the child can be evaluated, but the courts have held that, in the absence of other reasons supporting a finding against the mother with epilepsy, her condition cannot be the only reason for a negative finding.

As with all legal issues, women are advised to seek assistance from reputable counsel experienced in this particular area, i.e., family law, if they believe that they have been discriminated against because of their epilepsy or seizure disorder condition. Your local Epilepsy Foundation affiliate or bar association can make appropriate referrals to experienced, reputable attorneys in this area of the law.

Insurance

The area that has probably been least affected by the disability rights movement is the underwriting of health and life insurance. Unfortunately, however, whether a woman is insurable upon being diagnosed with epilepsy is often her most pressing concern. Many health insurance policies have requirements with respect to the nature or the length of exclusion for pre-existing conditions that adversely affect the insurability of individuals with epilepsy, e.g., requiring that an individual be an employee for 1 year prior to covering medical or hospitalization expenses arising from a health condition in existence upon the commencement of employment. Some insurance policies may contain permanent exclusions of coverage for pre-existing conditions.

It is not illegal under federal law, including the ADA, to have such a pre-existing condition requirement in an insurance policy as long as it is not used as a method to evade the purposes of the ADA. In addition, the ADA does not even require that an employer provide health insurance or other benefits, but if the employer chooses to offer insurance, an employee with a disability must be provided the same insurance benefits as all other employees similarly situated. The ADA also prohibits an employer from rejecting a job applicant with a disability or with a dependent who is disabled on the basis that the employer's insurance premiums will increase. In addition to federal law, the insurance commission of every state regulates and licenses each company that sells insurance within its boundaries. Therefore, these commissions are an appropriate place with which to lodge a complaint if you believe that your insurance company has discriminated against you wrongfully because of your epilepsy.

If your insurance company denies coverage for a medical or hospitalization expense connected with epilepsy, it is always advisable to pursue your right of appeal through the insurance company. Of course, most insurance companies now have 1–800 help lines and the individuals who respond can initially provide basic coverage information. However, if you have additional questions or the answers you receive are not satisfactory, ask for the department within the company responsible for reviewing coverage decisions, and speak directly with those individuals to ascertain if additional information from your physician would reverse the decision.

If you receive insurance through your employer and have no concerns regarding the confidentiality of your condition, contact your insurance representative or human resources designee within your employer organization to pursue your right of review. When I was first diagnosed with epilepsy, I had joined a law firm a few months earlier. The firm's insurance company initially denied coverage of my hospitalization and all medical expenses eventually resulting from my epilepsy on the basis of the pre-existing condition exclusion. Because I had been having complex partial seizures for 2 years prior to joining the firm (but was unaware of what they were and had not sought medical attention), the insurance company declared it was irrelevant that my initial diagnosis occurred after I had been employed for over 8 months. However, the human resources administrator within the firm, who was our contact with the insurance company, explained the facts of my hospitalization and, after providing a supporting letter from the attending neurologist, convinced the insurance underwriter to reverse its decision and cover my substantial hospitalization costs.

Although there may be no legal issue involved, as with some of the other areas discussed in this chapter, if you are denied insurance benefits because of your epilepsy, pursue the basis upon which you are denied and be satisfied that you have exhausted your remedies within the insurance underwriter and with your employer.

Conclusion

Women (and men) with epilepsy should not permit others to treat them socially in a fashion that suggests stereotypical beliefs or expectations, nor should they identify themselves in terms of their epilepsy. Similarly, they should not permit others to engage in discrimination against them or their children on the basis of their epilepsy, whether such action comes in the course of employment, child custody or adoption, or educational opportunities. Some reasonable restrictions may apply, such as those discussed in connection with driver's licensing laws and the reasonableness of accommodations required under the ADA.

However, if a woman believes she has been unlawfully discriminated against, she should record and document the treatment she receives to the best of her ability and seek the advice of a qualified attorney. The law, particularly the ADA, now guarantees rights to the disabled, but the strength of the remedies that will be won will only be as substantial as the energy with which the rights are pursued and exercised.

SELECTED REFERENCES

Epilepsy Foundation. *The Americans With Disabilities Act – A Guide to Provisions Affecting Persons With Seizure Disorders.* Landover, MD, 1992.

Wyllie Elaine. Legal aspects of epilepsy. In *The Treatment of Epilepsy: Principles and Practice,* 2nd edn. Williams and Wilkins, Baltimore, MD, 1997.

Epilepsy Foundation. *Seizure Disorders, Facts and Issues.* Landover, MD, 1998.

Cases

Eckles v. Consolidated Rail Corp., 94 F.3d 1041 (7th Cir. 1996.)

Jacques v. Clean-Up Group, 96 F.3d 506 (1st Cir. 1996.)

Martinson v. Kinney Shoe Corp., 104 F.3d 683 (4th Cir. 1997).

Matczak v. Frankford Candy and Chocolate Company, 136 F.3d 933 (3d Cir. 1997.)

Roberts by & Through Rodenberg-Roberts v. KinderCare Leaning Ctrs., 86 F.3d 844 (8th Cir. 1996.)

27

Work issues and epilepsy

Jim Troxell

Jim Troxell was formerly a member of the senior staff at the Epilepsy Foundation, where, among other things, he directed employment programs. Mr Troxell has been a strong supporter of the rights of people with epilepsy to be in the work force and has advocated for government-sponsored occupational training programs for people with epilepsy. The Epilepsy Foundation is now involved in a trial program with the Department of Labor to train people with epilepsy in new information technology. These skills enable people to have well-paid jobs from home – ideal for individuals without driver's licenses. Twenty-five percent of people with epilepsy are unemployed in a nation where the overall unemployment rate is 5%. Half say that their unemployment is directly related to seizures. I have heard stories of jobs lost in the executive office, in the classroom, in the shop, and from the assembly line because people were afraid of seizures. Certainly, any progress in employment nationwide requires education about epilepsy so that decisions about who can or cannot do the job are not made from ignorance. Each of us can do our small part by making certain that we provide accurate information about epilepsy to those around us and that we stand up against workplace discrimination whenever we see it.

MJM

Finding and keeping a job are a challenge for most people. Whether this involves a young adult's first job, making career changes, or seeking employment after the disappointment of layoff or termination, it takes a great deal of emotional energy and practical initiative to be successful.

In many developing countries, it is increasingly the case that everyone is expected to work – including women with young children. This social trend has come about rapidly in the past few decades and, because universal work is so new, the implications have not been fully recognized. Unique issues for women in the workforce include the need for more high-quality day care, more flexibility with leave time policies from employers, and more job training for women entering employment.

When both parents work, or when a single mother must work while raising her children, reliable day care is essential. If the extended family is not available, working women must find jobs with employers that offer day-care arrangements or must retain such services. Knowledge of these resources – how to select a provider, assessment of employer-provided benefits, how to arrange transportation to day care as well as to the place of employment – has become an essential consideration for working women.

Working full time and raising children demands more time, energy, and money than most parents have. This is difficult enough for a two-parent family with healthy children and enough money for adequate day care; a single parent with limited income can have real problems if her children are ill. Ideal jobs for women with dependents need to include some flexibility with hours, the ability to use personal sick leave to care for children, more part-time work, or stay-at-home jobs.

Many women who encounter situations in which employment becomes necessary – return to work after years of child-rearing, need for more personal income, or need to work in the absence of a partner's income – find they must go through a phase of pre-employment training to be equipped for the demands of the dynamic workplace of the twenty-first century. This may necessitate classroom/technical training or enrollment in a private or public sector job-training program. In either case, the individual is likely to encounter complicated application and eligibility procedures. It may take time and financial resources for a woman to become properly trained and educated for a suitable job.

Employment today typically requires flexibility, mastery of multiple skills, and willingness and ability to supplement employer-provided health benefits with a share of personal income. Part-time work has proliferated in recent years. Technological developments have increased the demand to use computers and sophisticated machinery. Fewer and fewer positions are available that provide lifetime employment at the same basic task(s) with fully paid benefits. In this new climate, most workers need to be resourceful and well suited to change.

Women with epilepsy who are working must confront the realities and dynamics of this contemporary environment while also living with the realities and dynamics of their condition. Despite advances in medical control, and regardless of the seizure type, frequency, or severity, most women with epilepsy encounter some degree of vocational difficulty. Before exploring specific facets of employment, it is helpful to examine factors common to the experience of epilepsy that make the disorder uniquely challenging.

Whereas employment success is clearly possible for women with epilepsy, the strategies to achieve it differ greatly for each individual, because people with seizure disorders have widely varied experience with the condition.

- Epilepsy is a *hidden, episodic* condition. For the majority of people, the challenges of living with epilepsy are not manifested through recognizable physical impairment. Only when the symptoms of epilepsy, typically unpredictable, periodically occur do most people with epilepsy appear to be disabled. This presents difficulties for those with underlying neurological or neuropsychological impairment because these aspects of epilepsy-related disability may be undiagnosed. It also presents difficulties for those who function without impairment as a general rule, but then experience a major disruption to the course of their daily living.
- The *spectrum of disability* associated with epilepsy is extraordinarily broad. The condition affects people with severe, multiple disability profiles as well as individuals who have no other difficulty with functional abilities. Seizure activity itself, because of seizure type, frequency, and manifestation, may be more or less challenging to personal functioning; the differences among individuals in the population are highly individualized.
- *Locus of control.* Seizures take away motor control and, in many cases, cause changes in consciousness. Treatment strategies may require lifestyle adjustments that compromise freedoms and choices; the side effects of the treatments may cause unwanted cognitive, physical, and emotional difficulties. Family members may overprotect loved ones with epilepsy to shield them from perceived physical harm or negative societal reactions.
- *Social stigma* may be a significant issue, especially if an individual experiences it directly because of family, peer, or cultural influences, among others. Individual self-esteem may be weakened if the person encounters negative reactions and barriers to independence and opportunity.

In consideration of these factors, the vocational experiences of women with epilepsy may be limited. Individuals with neuropsychological impairments are particularly vulnerable in an environment of fast-paced change. Occupations that require a high degree of adaptability may be closed to people with cognitive limitations or adjustment disorders. Memory deficits, language problems, and difficulties with perceptual–motor skills must all be taken into consideration.

The decision about whether or not to disclose epilepsy to an employer is especially sensitive. It is crucial that women who have seizure disorders understand their legal rights and responsibilities. These must be taken into consideration as they make decisions about whether and when to let an employer know about their condition. Of particular importance is a thorough assessment of whether epilepsy, and how it specifically affects the individual, has any bearing on whether it is possible for her to perform the essential demands of the job. If the seizure condition does not present barriers to the achievement of job responsibilities, it is probably neither necessary nor beneficial to disclose epilepsy. If some aspect of the disorder needs to be taken into consideration, such as work speed or memory difficulties, for example, it may be possible for the employer and employee to devise relatively simple strategies to compensate for those barriers. On the other hand, if the seizure condition presents significant problems with job performance or job safety, such that disability issues may not be accommodated, it is advisable that a different position be considered.

Given that many people with epilepsy report experiences with discrimination during the interviewing/selection process or after an employer learns of their condition, the decisions about disclosure must be considered very carefully. Misunderstanding and stigma can lead to unfair hiring practices and unfair treatment in the workplace.

Because locus of control and self-esteem are concerns for a large number of people with seizures, it is not uncommon for them to benefit greatly from professional counseling and peer interaction to address issues of concern. This support may involve in-depth psychological exploration or may simply involve building techniques for more confident interviewing skills and social interaction. As job seekers soon discover, a clear and self-assured presentation of skills is a key to success.

In view of these many complex issues, women with epilepsy will gain advantages with their employment efforts and career goals if they:

- Make a realistic assessment of their work skills and their seizure condition, considering the specific requirements of the job that is being sought.
- Seek professional support for a thorough assessment of neurological and neuropsychological factors that may need to be addressed when considering employment goals.

- Participate in specialized vocational preparation and/or occupational skills training services to develop interviewing skills, gain complete understanding of legal rights and responsibilities, learn job search techniques and new technical abilities.
- Make carefully considered judgments about when and how to disclose epilepsy, if disclosure is merited at all.

The vast majority of jobs are suitable for people with epilepsy. When a person possesses the right qualifications and experience, job suitability should normally be assumed. Blanket prohibitions should be avoided, and fair, individualized assessments should be made both of the demand of the work chosen and of the person with epilepsy concerned. Otherwise, such restrictions are discriminatory.

Other practical issues that must be explored include transportation, child care, and health benefits. A reliable means of getting to and from work is essential. Given that many people with epilepsy cannot accept employment that involves driving, public transportation or dependable ride sharing must be ensured. Women with epilepsy who have children need to be confident with their child-care arrangements so that time away from work is minimized. Finally, health insurance benefits must be carefully evaluated for cost, depth of coverage, and choice. Accepting employment that provides inadequate health benefits that do not provide for specialized care and consumer choice can have very bad results. Some women will need assistance with understanding the details of coverage and evaluating them relative to their personal and family medical needs.

Are there differences in the employment experiences of men and women with epilepsy? Although major differences are not clearly evident, some differences are notable when assessing data gathered on individuals served by the Epilepsy Foundation of America's National Employment Assistance Project in 1996–7.

Upon entering the program and reporting their experience with employment, women were more likely than men to have held their most recent job for less than 2 years (84.6% compared to 80.2%), to have been making less than $5.00 per hour (36.8% compared to 28.6%), and to have had a longer period of unemployment (over 2 years unemployed) than men (12.8% compared to 9%).

Success with job finding differs between the genders as well. Of the total number of males enrolled, 68% found employment, as compared with 61.5%

of the female participants. Whereas the same percentages of men and women could accept employment involving driving (65%) and chose to disclose their seizure condition to their employer (52%), other factors differed. Many more women found jobs in clerical, sales, and service positions (71.6%), which typically carry lower wage and benefit profiles, than men (55.6%). Indeed, female employees made less per hour for the jobs they took than males, and took jobs with fewer hours available per week.

Many women with seizure disorders are successfully employed. Having epilepsy does not prevent women from having successful jobs and careers. It is important, however, that careful decisions are made, that support is sought when it would be beneficial, and that qualifications and experience are promoted as the most important factors in a successful job search.

Note

A list of references/recommended reading on epilepsy and employment can be found in:

Chaplin J, Troxell J, Popovic M, Burke M, eds. *Recommended Reading List on Epilepsy and Employment.* International Bureau for Epilepsy, Heemstede, The Netherlands, 1995.

The Epilepsy Foundation's Campaign for Women's Health: bringing help and hope to women with epilepsy

Elizabeth A. Borda

A commitment to women

More than 1 million American women and girls are living with seizure disorders. Seizures and exposure to antiepileptic drugs (AEDs) alter female reproductive hormones and may have a negative effect on pregnancy and reproductive health. For instance, women with epilepsy are at greater risk for pregnancy complications, and fetal exposure to AEDs increases the risk of birth defects. The efficacy of hormonal contraceptives may be compromised by interactions with AEDs. Complicating these concerns, many women with epilepsy are seen by health-care professionals who are unfamiliar with these issues. A lack of research in this area compounds the problem.

For many years, the Epilepsy Foundation has received requests for information about the special issues facing women with epilepsy. In order to address these needs, the Foundation established a Committee on Women's Health. The committee included women with epilepsy, experts in the field of epilepsy and women's health, and representatives from the Food and Drug Administration and the National Institutes of Health. The committee was convened to explore these reports and identify the critical health issues facing women with epilepsy. It concluded that further research and better access to accurate information are needed to guide diagnosis, enhance medical care, and improve the quality of life for women who have seizures.

The committee made extensive recommendations in the areas of advocacy, public and professional education, patient care, and research and established objectives for a project focusing on the needs of women with epilepsy. As a result, the Women and Epilepsy Initiative was born.

As an important part of the Epilepsy Foundation's role in advocating for an improved quality of life for all people with seizure disorders, it is committed to addressing the unique health concerns of women with epilepsy. More comprehensive research focusing on the unique health concerns of women with epilepsy will provide information that ultimately improves their lives. Fundamental to this effort is a grassroots movement to promote and press for more attention to women's issues and a nationwide effort to educate health-care providers and the public and empower women with epilepsy and their families.

I have suffered with epilepsy for 30 years. My seizures always came just 5 days after the onset of my menstrual cycle. I wonder why so little research has been done on cases like mine? Such research is long overdue. I can't believe that I am the only woman who has experienced this. [E. Brown, Atlanta, GA.]

The mission

Given this background, the Epilepsy Foundation is committed to combating the unique problems of *all* women and girls with epilepsy through targeted research, improved medical care, and greater understanding in the community.

The goals

The Initiative has four primary goals.

- To empower women with epilepsy to improve their own health care by providing them with information and developing a network of mutual support to help them cope with the condition and its impact on their lives.

  I have put off starting a family in hopes that I can eventually be taken off [the drug] and be seizure free and drug free when I do become pregnant. This decision was very difficult for me. I know I need more support in this area. [L.A. Curley, Madison, WI.]

- To create awareness among health professionals of the unique difficulties confronting women with epilepsy and improve the medical and social services provided to women with the disorder through provider education.

How can I get my neurologist and gynecologist to quit bouncing me back and forth? [K. Miller, Sacramento, CA.]

- To improve public understanding of epilepsy, its impact on the lives of women and their families, and generate support for programs and services needed to assist them.

The judgement stated that the mother was 'unfit' because of her epilepsy. Use of epilepsy as a primary reason for taking someone's children away is morally, ethically, and legally wrong. I need help to clarify this for her and her attorney. [Social Worker assisting in child custody case, New Orleans, LA.]

- To stimulate scientific interest in the unique problems of women with epilepsy and generate support for research into the causes and solutions to these problems.

The lack of adequate scientific investigations into this important area is deplorable. [Robert J. Gumnit, MD, Director, Minnesota Comprehensive Epilepsy Program (MINCEP).]

The campaign

The Epilepsy Foundation's Women and Epilepsy Initiative is a campaign to bring hope and help to women with epilepsy. The project is divided into initiatives to break down community and institutional barriers.

The community initiative will provide the information and support that women with epilepsy need to work more effectively with their health-care providers to manage the effects of epilepsy in their daily lives.

It includes new informational, networking, and public awareness activities. Enhanced awareness of epilepsy and its impact on women will improve public understanding and help alleviate the psychological and social consequences that women with epilepsy face.

Information materials

- Information sheets on the specific issues that impact women with epilepsy, of which this handbook is an extension.

Community support

- Grants awarded in selected communities to Epilepsy Foundation affiliates to assist in the development of women's support and advocacy networks. Successful networks can be replicated throughout the nation.

National campaign for women's health

- A multimedia campaign to improve public understanding of epilepsy, its impact on the lives of women and their families, and to generate support for needed research and programs.
- The second phase of the campaign targets the scientific and provider communities. The goal is to stimulate scientific interest in the issues, generate support for research into causes and solutions, and sensitize and educate health-care providers about the difficulties confronting women with epilepsy.

Research support

- Direct support of research on issues affecting women with epilepsy.
- Advocate for increased governmental funding of gender-specific research in the public sector.

Provider education

- Develop educational materials and learning tools for health-care providers.

Health awareness

- A multifaceted campaign to raise awareness about the issues affecting women with epilepsy, especially targeting women's health-care providers.

Index

Note: page numbers in bold refer to tables and figures.